Urgent and Emergency Care of the Older Person

A Guide for Paramedics and Community Clinicians

Carol Robertson

and

Duncan Robertson

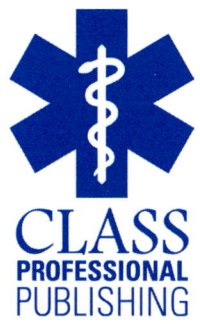

Class Professional Publishing have made every effort to ensure that the information, tables, drawings and diagrams contained in this book are accurate at the time of publication. The book cannot always contain all the information necessary for determining appropriate care and cannot address all individual situations; therefore, individuals using the book must ensure they have the appropriate knowledge and skills to enable suitable interpretation. Class Professional Publishing do not guarantee, and accept no legal liability of whatever nature arising from, or connected to, the accuracy, reliability, currency or completeness of the content of *Urgent and Emergency Care of the Older Person: A Guide for Paramedics and Community Clinicians*. Users must always be aware that such innovations or alterations after the date of publication may not be incorporated in the content. Please note, however, that Class Professional Publishing assume no responsibility whatsoever for the content of external resources in the text or accompanying online materials.

Text © Carol Robertson and Duncan Robertson 2025

All rights reserved. Without limiting the rights under copyright reserved above, no part of this publication may be reproduced, stored in or introduced into a retrieval system, or transmitted, in any form or by any means (electronic, mechanical, photocopying, recording or otherwise) without the prior written permission of the publisher of this book.

The information presented in this book is accurate and current to the best of the authors' knowledge.

The authors and publisher, however, make no guarantee as to, and assume no responsibility for, the correctness, sufficiency or completeness of such information or recommendation.

Printing history
This first edition printed in 2025, reprinted 2025.

The authors and publisher welcome feedback from the users of this book.
Please contact the publisher:

Class Professional Publishing,
The Exchange, Express Park, Bristol Road, Bridgwater, TA6 4RR
Telephone: 01278 472 800
Email: info@class.co.uk
Website: www.classprofessional.co.uk

Class Professional Publishing is an imprint of Class Publishing Ltd

A CIP catalogue record for this book is available from the British Library

Paperback ISBN: 9781859599860
ePub ISBN: 9781859599877
ePDF ISBN: 9781801611312

Cover design by Hybert Design

Designed and typeset by PHi Business Solutions

Printed in the UK by Short Run Press Limited

This book is printed on paper from responsible sources. Refer to local recycling guidance on disposal of this book.

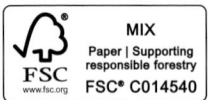

Product safety information can be found at https://www.classprofessional.co.uk/terms-of-use/gpsr-statement/

Dedicated to the memory of Connie and Fred Entwistle.

And to inspire our futures,
Milly Robertson, Tom Robertson,
Oliver Entwistle and Ophelia Entwistle.

The College of Paramedics is dedicated to advancing the profession and supporting paramedics at every stage of their careers. This series of texts, written specifically for paramedics, cover a wide range of topics that will benefit any member of the profession from pre-registration learner to seasoned practitioner. Addressing many of the knotty subject areas that paramedics face in their work, the series is written for paramedics across a variety of roles and sectors.

Developed by subject matter experts, these accessible, evidence-based resources align closely with the College of Paramedics' curriculum guidance, supporting pre-registration learners in meeting the professional expectations of the role. Whether used as a reference guide to reinforce knowledge or as a leisurely read to explore complex subjects, these books are a welcome addition to any paramedic's collection.

Paramedic Research: Principles, Designs and Methods

Edited by Julia Williams, Graham McClelland

Urgent and Emergency Care of the Older Person - A Guide for Paramedics and Community Clinicians

By Carol Robertson, Duncan Robertson

The Wellbeing and Resilience Workbook for Ambulance Clinicians

By Laura Simmons, Blaire Morgan, Joanne Mildenhall

Decision Making in Paramedic Practice

Edited by Andy Collen

Law and Ethics for Paramedics: An Essential Guide

Edited by Georgette Eaton

Primary Care for Paramedics

By Georgette Eaton, Alyesha Proctor, Joseph St Leger-Francis

Mental Health Care in Paramedic Practice

By Ursula Rolfe, David Partlow

Contents

About the Editors — vii
Contributors — ix
Acknowledgements — xiii
Abbreviations — xv

Introduction — 1
Carol Robertson and Duncan Robertson

Chapter 1 Theories and Physiology of Ageing — 7
Asangaedem Akpan

Chapter 2 Person-Centred Communication — 19
Gemma Howlett

Chapter 3 Frailty — 31
Carol Robertson and Tom Mallinson

Chapter 4 Long-Term Conditions — 49
Tom Mallinson

Chapter 5 Mental Health and Cognition — 65
Axel Laurell, Viveca Kirthisingha and Benjamin Underwood

Chapter 6 Polypharmacy and Medicines Review — 81
Ruth Harris and Gavin Ronaldson

Chapter 7 Activities of Daily Living — 103
Sophie Wallington and Beverley Clare

Chapter 8 Falls — 119
Carol Robertson

Contents

Chapter 9   **Major Trauma**   141
Duncan Robertson

Chapter 10   **Palliative and End-of-Life Care**   155
Edward O'Brian

Chapter 11   **Social Care**   173
Charlotte Walker and Peter Gosling

Chapter 12   **Safeguarding**   185
Gwenan Jones-Parry and Nikki Harvey

Index   201

About the Editors

Carol Robertson is an Advanced Clinical Practitioner and paramedic. She works at East Cheshire NHS Trust within the Older Persons Assessment and Liaison (OPAL) team following a long career with the North West Ambulance Service. She holds an MSc in Advanced Clinical Practice including a module in Care of the Older Frail Adult. She contributed two chapters, 'Delirium and Dementia' and 'Older People' to *Mental Health Care in Paramedic Practice* by Ursula Rolfe and David Partlow. She recently reviewed the paramedic modules: 'Why Falls and Frailty Matter' and 'Falls assessment and management for paramedics' for Health Education England's eLearning for Health. Furthermore, she has delivered podcasts on older adults plus two College of Paramedics CPD webinars, 'Older Adults and Frailty' and 'Delirium'. Carol strives to encourage healthcare colleagues to find an interest in caring for older people. She enjoys caring for older patients and loves to hear their stories. Carol is married to Duncan and their lives revolve around their dogs!

Duncan Robertson is an experienced paramedic leader who has worked in a number of roles within UK ambulance services. He started his career in Greater Manchester (North West Ambulance Service), moving to the Welsh Ambulance Services University NHS Trust in 2018 as a consultant paramedic. He is currently the Chief Paramedic Officer for South Central Ambulance Service NHS Foundation Trust where he started in September 2024. Duncan was one of the team that contributed to the 2017 *JRCALC Clinical Guidelines* chapter on Falls in Older Adults and undertook a qualitative study on frailty as part of his Master's in Clinical Research dissertation. He has a professional interest in the care provided for older adults by ambulance clinicians and is keen that the individuality and complexity of these important members of our patient cohort are acknowledged and acted upon to provide the best levels of care. Duncan has two children, Milly and Tom, and is married to Carol.

Contributors

Asangaedem Akpan graduated from the College of Medicine, University of Ibadan, Nigeria in 1992. He is a recipient of the UK NHS Clinical Excellence Awards for service developments and contribution to medical education. He has 30 years' experience as a medical doctor on three continents with experience of population health approaches to planning well-being and health. In July of 2023, he was appointed UN International Consultant for Older People working with the National Senior Citizens Centre in Nigeria to develop minimum standards of care for older people. He is now based in Western Australia as a Consultant Geriatrician at Bunbury Regional Hospital, Adjunct Associate Professor at the University of Western Australia and Adjunct Clinical Associate Professor in the Medical School of Curtin University. He has several peer reviewed publications and has contributed to chapters in medical textbooks, received research grants and supervised PhD students. He can be found on LinkedIn and X (@asanakpan).

Edward O'Brian began his career as an Emergency Medical Technician in London Ambulance Service in 2002. He holds a degree in paramedic science and a Master's degree in palliative medicine. He is a palliative care paramedic and the clinical lead for palliative care at Welsh Ambulance Services University NHS Trust. Edward has developed and introduced multiple new ways of working within the ambulance service in Wales to better support patients who are receiving end-of-life care: these include the introduction of just in case medications onto every ambulance; the introduction of an end-of-life care rapid transport service to convey dying patients to their preferred place of death without delay; a 'Wish Ambulance' service staffed by volunteers from across the Trust to help dying patients experience a meaningful journey; and the introduction of the UK's first rotational palliative care paramedics.

Beverley Clare is an Advanced Clinical Practitioner working in Manchester Local Care Organisation Community Services within Manchester University NHS Foundation Trust. She currently works alongside Sophie Wallington with whom she co-authored Chapter 7 of this book. In 2007, she graduated from the University of Salford as an Occupational Therapist and went on to complete a postgraduate diploma in Accessible and Inclusive Design of the Built Environment in 2014. Later that year she joined Manchester Local Care Organisation Community Services as a Senior Occupational Therapist working alongside North West Ambulance Service, general practice, secondary care and care homes before embarking on the MSc in Advanced Clinical Practice, graduating in 2019. Beverley has numerous specialist interests;

in particular the built environment, housing and their influence on health, in addition to frailty, dementia and delirium. Beverley has guest lectured at the University of Bolton for the frailty module and offered some support to the development of the Advanced Care of the Frail Older Adult as an honorary lecturer and external examiner at Manchester Metropolitan University.

Peter Gosling is a retired social worker with over 35 years' experience of working in adult social care services. Having qualified with a Master's degree at Manchester University in 1988, Peter was involved in setting up one of the early pilot schemes for care management, following the implementation of the NHS and Community Care Act 1990. In 2001, Peter won a national Health and Social Care Award for a multidisciplinary service focussed on facilitating hospital discharge. Peter has managed home care and care home services as well as social work, occupational therapy and mental health services in several north-west authorities. He has also delivered training for social care staff in a variety of settings and completed a Diploma in Management Studies. From 2014 to 2022, he was Head of Service in East Cheshire with a particular interest in supporting social care services working in two busy hospitals.

Nikki Harvey is a Registered General Nurse with an MSc in Child Protection. She was the Head of Safeguarding for the Welsh Ambulance Services University NHS Trust (WAST) at the time of writing, a position she held since 2017. Nikki has over 20 years' experience working collaboratively within the safeguarding and public protection arena in a variety of health service settings. On behalf of WAST, Nikki has been instrumental in the development and implementation of a digital safeguarding reporting system which is now in use across Wales. Nikki has been influential in strategic safeguarding, chairing the National Ambulance Safeguarding Assurance Group (NASAG) for several years. Having recently retired early, part of Nikki's legacy will be the impact of her revolutionary safeguarding reporting in WAST.

Ruth Harris is an Advanced Clinical Practitioner, working in the Ageing and Complex Medicine department at Salford Care Organisation. Ruth enjoys a split role, providing same-day emergency care to older people living with frailty that present to the emergency department and specialist in-reach into the Peri-Operative Care of Older People Undergoing General Surgery. She also holds an Honorary Clinical Lecturer position at Manchester Metropolitan University, contributing to the teaching of trainee advanced clinical practitioners and nursing students. She is a Pharmacist by discipline and graduated with a Master's in Pharmacy (MPharm (Hons)) from the University of Manchester, after which she achieved a Postgraduate Diploma in Clinical Pharmacy from Liverpool John Moores University. She has acquired extensive experience in the care of older adults across the healthcare landscape before going on to complete a Master's in Advanced Clinical Practice at Manchester Metropolitan University. Ruth lives in Manchester with her husband and two very spoiled cats.

Gemma Howlett is the Head of Teaching, Learning and Student Experience in the Institute of Health at University of Cumbria and is a registered paramedic. Gemma holds an FdSc in Pre-Hospital, Unscheduled and Emergency Care from the University of Worcester, a BSc (Hons) in Sport and Exercise Science from the University of

Gloucestershire, a PGCert in Learning and Teaching from the University of Worcester and a Master's in Advanced Clinical Practice from the University of Worcester. Gemma is reading for her PhD at Lancaster University in the School of Justice and Education. Gemma's PhD is looking at sexual harassment in UK ambulance services. Gemma is a Senior Fellow with the Higher Education Academy. Her research interests are in equality, diversity and inclusion and widening participation in paramedic practice, gender equality, gender pay gaps, gender disparity in senior management roles in higher education and Ambulance Services.

Gwenan Jones-Parry MSc, BSc (Hons), DipHE Paramedic Science, Senior Safeguarding Specialist, Welsh Ambulance Services University NHS Trust (WAST). Gwenan worked as a paramedic in South Wales before specialising and joining the Safeguarding Team. Contributing to strategic and operational safeguarding, providing safeguarding advice to colleagues, attending multi-agency safeguarding forums and developing safeguarding training are all part of her daily role. Gwenan has been a key part in the work to digitalise the safeguarding reporting process in WAST, making safeguarding reports more accessible to colleagues and the reporting process more efficient.

Viveca Kirthisingha is a Fellow of the Royal College of Physicians, London with an interest in Education. She has been a Consultant Community Geriatrician at Cambridgeshire and Peterborough NHS Foundation Trust and an Honorary Consultant in Elderly Care at Cambridge University Hospitals NHS Foundation Trust since 2008. She is the Undergraduate Tutor for final year medical students in 'Medicine in the Community' as part of their Acute Medicine block. She has an interest in optimising care for all patients including those with mental health conditions. She works on physical health wards and in care homes and provides an in-reach model of care to old age psychiatry wards in Cambridge.

Axel Laurell is a Specialty Trainee in Old-Age Psychiatry at Cambridgeshire and Peterborough NHS Foundation Trust and a Clinical Research Associate at the University of Cambridge. He studied medicine (MBChB) and neuroscience (MSc) at the University of Dundee, graduating in 2019. After completing the Academic Foundation Programme in Edinburgh, he moved to Cambridge as an National Institute for Health and Care Research Academic Clinical Fellow to start his specialty training in psychiatry. Axel is a Member of the Royal College of Psychiatrists (MRCPsych) and has also completed the Postgraduate Certificate in Medical Education (PGCertMedEd). He is currently undertaking a 3-year PhD fellowship at the University of Cambridge where he is using clinical and neuroimaging data from cohort studies to improve our understanding of the symptoms and progression of dementia.

Tom Mallinson began his career with the London Ambulance Service NHS Trust. He then read Medicine at Warwick Medical School and undertook further education in primary care, wilderness medicine and healthcare education. He is a fellow of the Royal Geographical Society, the Higher Education Academy and the Faculty of Remote, Rural and Humanitarian Healthcare of the Royal College of Surgeons of Edinburgh. Tom has published primary research and educational materials and is a senior lecturer with the College of Remote and Offshore Medicine. Tom lives in the Scottish Highlands with his wife, dog, chickens and flock of grumpy Hebridean sheep.

Contributors

Gavin Ronaldson is the Primary Care Network Lead Pharmacist for Better Health MCR, which provides primary care services for around 44,000 patients in Central Manchester. They have extensive experience of working in older persons care in both primary and secondary care and have completed several postgraduate qualifications including an MSc in Advanced Clinical Practice. In addition to their clinical role, they also work as an honorary lecturer at Manchester Metropolitan University, teaching students on the Advanced Care of the Frail and Older Adult module on medicines use and deprescribing in older adults living with frailty. Outside of work, they enjoy spending time with friends and family and walking their dog, George.

Benjamin Underwood studied natural science at Oxford University and medicine in London. He completed his psychiatric training in Cambridge, including a PhD in molecular neurogenetics. He is currently an associate professor in applied and translational old age psychiatry at the University of Cambridge and honorary consultant psychiatrist at Cambridgeshire and Peterborough NHS Foundation Trust (CPFT). He is research and development director at CPFT, clinical lead for dementia in the East of England for the Clinical Research Network and national Clinical Research Network lead for stratified medicine in dementia.

Charlotte Walker started work in Queen Alexandra's Royal Army Nursing Corps serving in the UK, Cyprus and Oman. She then worked for Age Concern Swansea as an Operational Manager with responsibility for integrated care services. When promoted to Assistant Director, Charlotte's interests expanded into local government and health boards. In 2008 she was successful in being appointed into social services and led on many key areas, including day care and residential services. Charlotte was then seconded to an integrated care role as an Assistant Locality Manager which soon became a permanent post and enabled her to lead on setting up the first community resource team in Wales. This work also enabled her to achieve an MSc in Public Health and Partnerships in Care. After 12 years in Local Authority she moved to work for the Welsh Ambulance Services University NHS Trust (WAST) as the Older Persons Lead. She worked with a mixed team of individuals to develop the Older Persons Strategy in WAST. She is currently Senior Quality Lead for WAST.

Sophie Wallington is a clinical academic, working as an Advanced Clinical Practitioner (ACP)/Clinical Lead for Manchester Local Care Organisation Community Services, within Manchester University NHS Foundation Trust. She holds a BSc (Hons) in Physiotherapy from the University of Liverpool, an MSc Advanced Practice from the University of Bolton and a Postgraduate Certificate in Education from Manchester Metropolitan University. In her clinical role as an ACP she works closely with the Northwest Ambulance Service, rapidly responding to patients in acute health or social care crisis and managing highly complex frail patients out of hospital. Here she works closely alongside Beverley Clare, with whom she has co-authored Chapter 7 of this book. Alongside this role, Sophie is a Senior Lecturer at Manchester Metropolitan University, Unit Lead for the Advanced Care of the Frail and Older Person Unit, part of the ACP Apprenticeship MSc.

Acknowledgements

We would like to thank all authors for the expertise and generosity of their contributions. Their dedication and willingness while working in demanding health and social care environments has been inspiring. Thank you.

To Katherine Totterdell from Class Professional Publishing for her constant support and encouragement from conception to publication.

Thank you to the Robertsons: Milly, Tom, Lorna and Duncan (snr), Stuart, Eve, Emma and William who have championed our voyage of discovery as editors and listened to our ideas with unwavering encouragement.

Thank you to the Entwistles: Tina, Paul, Oliver and Ophelia for giving us the space and time to develop this book.

Thank you to Carol Robinson for posing for the photographs in Chapter 8: Falls and for her encouragement throughout. Thank you to Wendy and Kay Walsh for the cover photographs.

A special thank you to Caroline, Kirstie and Mike and all of our friends who have listened to us and allowed our thoughts, ideas and progress to be woven into our social events.

Stephanie Narey and the Older Persons Assessment and Liaison staff within the East Chesire NHS Trust for their constant support.

The contributions of the reviewers and the College of Paramedics.

To Pippy and Teddy, our dogs, who have sacrificed cuddles, walks and being fed on time, thank you!

Lastly, but most importantly, to all of our patients and their families who have put faith in our knowledge, skills and abilities in their time of crisis, thank you.

Abbreviations

4AT	4 'A's Test
ACP	advanced clinical practitioner
ACB	anticholinergic burden
ADLs	activities of daily living
ADR	adverse drug reaction
AFib	atrial fibrillation
AMHP	approved mental health practitioner
AS	aortic stenosis
ATLS	Advanced Trauma Life Support
BGS	British Geriatrics Society
bpm	beats per minute
CBT	cognitive behavioural therapy
CFS	Clinical Frailty Scale
CGA	comprehensive geriatric assessment
CK	creatine kinase
COPD	chronic obstructive pulmonary disease
CRP	C-reactive protein
DOAC	direct oral anticoagulants
ECG	electrocardiogram
ECT	electroconvulsive therapy
ED	emergency department
FAST	face, arms, speech, time
FBC	full blood count
GCS	Glasgow Coma Scale
GP	general practitioner
HECTOR	Heartlands Elderly Care Trauma & Ongoing Recovery
ISS	Injury Severity Score
JRCALC	Joint Royal Colleges Ambulance Liaison Committee

Abbreviations

LGBTQIA+	lesbian, gay, bisexual, transgender, queer (or questioning), intersex, and asexual (or allies)
LTC	long-term condition
MDT	multidisciplinary team
MHRA	Medicines and Healthcare products Regulatory Agency
MI	myocardial infarction
MTC	major trauma centre
NEWS2	National Early Warning Score 2
NHS	National Health Service
NHSE	NHS England
NOF	neck of femur
NSAID	non-steroidal anti-inflammatory drug
OA	osteoarthritis
OH	orthostatic hypotension
OHID	Office for Health Improvement and Disparities
OTC	over the counter
PEFR	peak expiratory flow rate
POC	package of care
PPC	preferred place of care
PPD	preferred place of death
RCP	Royal College of Physicians
ROM	range of motion
RPS	Royal Pharmaceutical Society
RTC	road traffic collision
SAIL	Secure Anonymised Information Linkage
SCIE	Social Care Institute for Excellence
SDEC	same-day emergency care
STS	sit-to-stand
TARN	Trauma Audit and Research Network
TIA	transient ischaemic attack
TFT	thyroid function test
TUGT	Timed Up and Go Test
U&E	urea and electrolytes
UCR	urgent community response
WAST	Welsh Ambulance Services University NHS Trust
WHO	World Health Organization

Introduction

Carol Robertson and Duncan Robertson

Setting the Scene

The number of older adults in the UK is increasing as the generation born after the second world war, sometimes known as 'Baby Boomers', enter retirement age (Office for National Statistics (ONS), 2018 and 2023a). Despite stories in the media about the 'burden' of old age, what we are largely seeing is a societal success due to significant changes in the quality of healthcare, housing (The Health Foundation, 2024), education (Age UK, 2011), diet and nutrition (GOV.UK, 2017) and, despite the recent cost of living crisis, an overall increase in population wealth, albeit increasingly unequally divided (ONS, 2021). As a result of this demographic shift, we are seeing a commensurate increase in the number of older people requiring help to maintain their health and independence compared with earlier generations, with existing services having to adapt as a consequence.

The World Health Organization (WHO) highlights that although people are living longer, healthy years have remained similar to previous decades, indicating more years of poorer health (WHO, 2022). So, while there are overall patterns of improvement, structural inequalities still remain. It is also significant that those who are the most vulnerable or deprived are also the most likely to have poorer health outcomes, poorer education, poorer housing and poorer diet. These are the patterns that follow individuals into older age and provide the context for the care we are asked to deliver.

Despite the progress made, there remain deep divisions in wealth and deprivation across the population and this plays out in health and social care. It is therefore important for us to not stereotype the older generation, to actively look for the individual and to listen to their stories. Older people may not see themselves as old and may want to present themselves as able to cope better than they may realistically be able to. Theirs is not a life defined by walking sticks or walking frames, ageing or comorbidities, but one that demonstrates adaptations to their newly adjusted lifeworld. With this in mind, as clinicians, we need to adapt how we communicate with this diverse group, to better understand their needs and requirements, their fears and vulnerabilities and their hopes and goals. If we do not make efforts to understand, empathise and relate, we run the risk of paternalism and control as decisions made at the point of care are likely to be made to suit our own internal biases.

Introduction

Therefore, to understand older people, it is helpful to move away from simply using biological age and take a deeper look at the individual and their circumstances. We must recognise that the individuals who access health and social services are a subset of the overall older population. As such, notions of old age starting at 65 should be challenged. The increase in UK state retirement age to 66 and then to 67 between 2026 and 2028 means this cut off is largely an artificial construct. There are robust and healthy individuals living very well into their nineties, while centenarians are also increasing in number (ONS, 2023b). Though there are increasing numbers of robust elders, we also see the 'younger old', often in deprived areas, living with multiple comorbidities and with frailty. There also remain marginalised communities of older adults who we see in practice – we need to further understand, and adapt our approaches to, these communities.

This diversity, along with clinical and social complexity, means there is no one-size-fits-all approach to providing high-quality care (NHS, 2019). Unlike younger people, the model of single system issues does not readily apply and the complexity that will be encountered when providing care for older people is highlighted within the chapters of this book. With the increase in this cohort of patients comes the need to draw some of the learning together and to deepen our understanding, making us better clinicians. We are aiming to bring more knowledge to readers and students so that we can better prepare ourselves to provide excellent care for our largest patient population.

Throughout this book, we encourage readers to practice holistically, to consider the individual patient, their circumstances, their wishes and needs. We increasingly recognise that traditional ambulance practice, dominated by rapid assessment and transfer to hospital, no longer applies. Older people are vulnerable and at risk in hospital, with the consequences of a long stay being bed-bound patients who experience subsequent deconditioning followed by an increased risk of falls with injury or hospital acquired infection, which further accelerates the deconditioning process. As a result, the decisions we make at scene or in the community can have far reaching consequences, both positive and negative.

Wherever possible we encourage the use of remote senior clinical support to enable shared decision making or early calls to the specialists who may already be involved in providing care for the patient. The wishes of the patient and their family should be introduced at an early stage. Record keeping is an important aspect of care, so do not underestimate the importance of the ambulance or community record to those who provide care further along the pathway. Insights gleaned on scene, or in the patient's home, can play an important part in the ongoing care or discharge later.

The Book

This book aims to demonstrate the principles that underpin improvements to our provision of care for older people which involves the multidisciplinary team (MDT) approach. Delivering holistic, personalised care will enable individuals to stay well and live independently at home for as long as possible. We must listen to and support what the person's needs and wishes are, especially towards the end of their lives, and to support older people with health issues to remain close to home (NHS, 2023). The British Geriatrics Society (BGS, 2023) highlight that annual frailty expenditure within UK healthcare systems amounts to approximately £5.8 billion. This may be reduced with correct prevention and care which they remark can be provided by primary and community-based care. For older people, such a proactive approach can greatly decrease emergency hospital admissions (BGS, 2023). Furthermore, NHS Confederation state that:

> *'community and primary care providers working together will be central to achieving national ambitions to support more people with frailty to live well at or closer to home. The sector plays a key role at every stage of the frailty care pathway: in prevention, crisis response and intermediate care.'*
>
> (NHS Confederation, 2024)

We have asked a range of experts (our very own MDT), including those with a developed interest, from within medicine, social care, paramedicine and therapies to contribute their expertise to this book.

We begin with an overview of ageing theories to set the scene and then build on this to consider communication with older people. Also underpinning common clinical presentations is Chapter 3: Frailty. The following chapters explore and explain commonly encountered scenarios and presentations. The information provided in each chapter is not a protocol or flowchart, but pertinent to aid the formulation of your plan of care. Our content is aimed at a range of clinical environments that paramedics find themselves working in, both within and outside of the ambulance world.

There are sections to help those new to, or developing their practice, from undergraduate and newly qualified, to those looking at roles with extended, specialist and advanced practice. This text highlights clinical complexity and breaks away from the single systems model often taught at undergraduate level. As a result, you will notice referral to other chapters demonstrating the connecting challenges for older people, and this is deliberate. Readers are encouraged to make their own connections too. Single systems are reinforced by how health, and secondary care in particular, is structured into specialties. General practice, the primary care MDT, community services and geriatricians increasingly provide a generalist overview with the patient at the centre of the decision-making process, and the following chapters will enable a range of community-based clinicians to be able to contribute to the care of this group of patients.

For undergraduates, this text provides a necessary oversight to the common aspects of care that will be frequently encountered both on placement and when newly qualified. The sixth edition of the College of Paramedics' pre-registration Paramedic Curriculum specifically includes having knowledge in the care of older people (College of Paramedics, 2024) which this text will support. For those looking to develop towards advanced practice, the chapters aim to give an overview, but have a wealth of material to refer to, to encourage you to read further and develop a depth of knowledge. For those established in their practice, we hope that the content provides

Introduction

new information to improve practice and to contribute to continuing professional development and re-registration or re-validation.

Each of these chapters could be a book in its own right, so the reader is encouraged to follow up on the key resources and references to deepen their own knowledge.

Language

A note about language – you will see that we do not use the term 'elderly' or 'the elderly' (unless within a quote, test, title or reference). There is a great deal of debate in terms of the words we use as some of the language of the past is steeped in ageism, often creating a barrier to healthcare (Falconer and O'Neill 2007, Hekmat-Panah 2019). Terms like 'elderly', as argued by David Oliver (2015) 'reduce everyone from sixty-five to one-hundred years into a single amorphous (vulnerable, dependent and invisible) mass'. We have made a deliberate choice to use terms such as older person or older adult, as this represents a kinder, more inclusive approach. Similarly, we do not advocate for the use of frailty or dementia as a label or as something to be suffering with. These are terms and diagnoses that people live with and as such may have to make adaptations for, but it does not define them. It is increasingly recognised that terms which were previously used are now seen as pejorative and, if used in practice or in front of patients, may lead to a disconnect and break in trust between patient and professional. There is stigma attached to many terms associated with ageing. We have tried to consider these in the text and would encourage you to do the same in practice.

Lastly, we hope you enjoy this book and that it helps to deepen your understanding and knowledge of caring for older people. Mostly, we hope it ignites a passion to care, appreciate and listen to the stories of older people. Remember, these are your grandparents, parents – and it will one day be you too!

References

Age UK (2011). Healthy ageing evidence review. Available at: https://www.ageuk.org.uk/globalassets/age-uk/documents/reports-and-publications/reports-and-briefings/health--wellbeing/rb_april11_evidence_review_healthy_ageing.pdf [accessed 28th September 2023].

British Geriatrics Society (BGS) (2023). Protecting the rights of older people to health and social care. British Geriatrics Society statement, supported by RCP London and RCP Edinburgh. Available at: https://www.bgs.org.uk/policy-and-media/protecting-the-rights-of-older-people-to-health-and-social-care [accessed 28th September 2023].

College of Paramedics (2024). Paramedic curriculum (6th edition). Available at: https://collegeofparamedics.co.uk/COP/ProfessionalDevelopment/Developing%20a%20New%20Paramedic%20Curriculum.aspx [accessed 2nd June 2024].

Falconer M, O'Neill D (2007). Out with 'the old', elderly, and aged. *British Medical Journal*, 334(7588): 316.

GOV.UK (2017). Helping older people maintain a healthy diet: a review of what works. Available at: https://www.gov.uk/government/publications/helping-older-people-maintain-a-healthy-diet-a-review-of-what-works/helping-older-people-maintain-a-healthy-diet-a-review-of-what-works [accessed 29th September 2024].

Health Foundation (2024). Evidence hub: What drives health inequalities? Available at: https://www.health.org.uk/evidence-hub [accessed 27th September 2023].

Hekmat-Panah J (2019). 'Elderly' – an outdated and potentially harmful term. *British Medical Journal Opinion*. Available at: https://blogs.bmj.com/bmj/2019/03/01/javad-hekmat-panahelderly-outdated-potentially-harmful-term/ [accessed 28th September 2024].

NHS (2019). The NHS long term plan. Available at: https://www.longtermplan.nhs.uk/wp-content/uploads/2019/08/nhs-long-term-plan-version-1.2.pdf [accessed 2nd May 2024].

NHS (2023). Ageing well. Available at: https://www.longtermplan.nhs.uk/areas-of-work/ageing-well/ [accessed 28th September 2023].

NHS Confederation (2024). Supporting people living with frailty. Available at: https://www.nhsconfed.org/publications/supporting-people-frailty#:~:text=Community%20and%20primary%20care%20providers,crisis%20response%20and%20intermediate%20care [accessed 12th April 2024].

Office for National Statistics (ONS) (2018). Living longer: how our population is changing and why it matters. Available at: https://www.ons.gov.uk/peoplepopulationandcommunity/birthsdeathsandmarriages/ageing/articles/livinglongerhowourpopulationischangingandwhyitmatters/2018-08-13 [accessed 2nd May 2024].

Office for National Statistics (ONS) (2021). Household total wealth in Great Britain: April 2018 to March 2020. Available at: https://www.ons.gov.uk/peoplepopulationandcommunity/personalandhouseholdfinances/incomeandwealth/bulletins/distributionofindividualtotalwealthbycharacteristicingreatbritain/april2018tomarch2020#:~:text=Median%20total%20wealth%20for%20individuals,of%20wealth%20across%20the%20population [accessed 28th September 2024].

Office for National Statistics (ONS) (2023a). Profile of the older population living in England and Wales in 2021 and changes since 2011. Available at: https://www.ons.gov.uk/peoplepopulationandcommunity/birthsdeathsandmarriages/ageing/articles/profileoftheolderpopulationlivinginenglandandwalesin2021andchangessince2011/2023-04-03 [accessed 28th September 2023].

Office for National Statistics (ONS) (2023b). Centenarians living in England and Wales in 2021. Available at: https://www.ons.gov.uk/peoplepopulationandcommunity/birthsdeathsandmarriages/ageing/articles/centenarianslivinginenglandandwalesin2021/2023-09-18#:~:text=On%20Census%20Day%20in%202021,as%20life%20expectancy%20has%20improved [accessed 27th September 2023].

Oliver D (2015). Minding our language around care for older people and why it matters. *British Medical Journal Opinion*. Available at: https://blogs.bmj.com/bmj/2015/05/07/david-oliver-minding-our-language-around-care-for-older-people/ [accessed 28th September 2023].

World Health Organization (WHO) (2022). Ageing and health. Available at: https://www.who.int/news-room/fact-sheets/detail/ageing-and-health [accessed 1st June 2024].

Chapter 1

Theories and Physiology of Ageing

Asangaedem Akpan

> **Learning Points**
>
> This chapter will provide the theoretical underpinnings to the remainder of the book. At the end of this chapter, you will:
>
> - Understand the multiple approaches to ageing theories
> - Understand that biological processes are not linear and not easily transferable across groups from diverse backgrounds
> - Understand how ageing manifests in multiple systems within the body.

Introduction

Ageing is associated with a progressive decline in capacity and capability to conduct activities of daily living (ADLs). This decline is variable across individuals, groups and the world. This variation results in individuals who remain reasonably fit and well throughout most of their lives while others develop several conditions which impact their functioning. The factors that contribute to these are both intrinsic and extrinsic. The intrinsic factors relate to genetics and specific conditions that people acquire while extrinsic factors are related to the determinants of well-being and health which impact all human beings from birth until death.

There are over 300 theories (Lipsky and King 2015) which have been postulated to explain ageing. This number continues to increase as research reveals potentially better explanations. Just like a jigsaw puzzle there will be some pieces missing and our understanding will remain incomplete. However, we have enough of the jigsaw puzzle pieces to have a reasonably good working knowledge of ageing. This serves as a foundation upon which further discoveries and explanations can be built.

Biological Theories of Ageing

Free Radical Theory

The most popular and well known is Harman's free radical theory of ageing (Harman, 1956). The human cell produces free radicals from oxidation and these radicals are counterbalanced by an antioxidant system. In ageing the free radical production is more than the antioxidant system can cope with. The excess free radicals are toxic and damage the cell. The process of free radical production is also referred to as oxidation. Research has confirmed that older animals have more oxidation occurring than young animals (Stadtman, 1992). Excess free radicals have been associated with certain conditions (Harman, 1978) and administering specific antioxidants has been shown to increase the lifespan (Varela-López et al., 2023). While this was a popular theory, evidence is increasingly being discovered which questions it (Speakman and Selman, 2011).

Genetic Theory

The genetic theory of ageing involves damage to mitochondrial genes and DNA. Chronic oxidative stress damages portions of the DNA. Most damaged portions are repaired, but the unrepaired portions accumulate with ageing which is toxic (Chaudhary et al., 2023). Mitochondria are the source of energy in cells in the form of adenosine triphosphate. They have a significant impact on skeletal muscle ageing; however, if these processes are not counterbalanced, there is a gradual reduction in muscle fibres and sarcopenia develops.

Genetic theories of ageing are derived from cross-species studies. There are varying ideas in terms of how genetics contribute to ageing, but it is generally acknowledged as not being the sole cause or reason for ageing. Key ideas include the accumulation of minor genetic mutations caused by damage to portions of DNA that remain unrepaired which may contribute to ageing at a cellular level; the late effects of specific genes, whereby there is a balance between reproduction and mortality as genes with protective mechanisms early in life contribute to increased mortality in later, or non-productive years; and the environmental adaptations whereby a lack of hazards that interfere with life expectancy lead to an increase in the number of those with adaptive mutations that directly lead to a slowing of the ageing process. As a result, there is no single dominant genetic theory of ageing.

Adaptive Homeostasis Theory

The adaptive homeostasis theory of ageing has been claimed to address some of the shortcomings in the free radical theory of ageing (Pomatto et al., 2018). The decline associated with ageing is proposed to result from a reduced ability of the mechanisms of homeostasis in the body to adapt to temporary changes in the stress protective systems. It does not regard the production of excess free radicals as a binary process. It explains that this process is more dynamic and fluctuates from minutes to hours, days and months.

The Epigenetic Clock Theory

The epigenetic clock theory of ageing is a more objective way of utilising biological rather than chronological age markers to understand the capability of a person across the life course and the changes that occur in those capabilities with getting older (Hovarth and Raj, 2018). While chronological age counts the time from birth, biological age takes account of a person's physiological state. Accurate biomarkers of ageing needed to be identified for this to work. This was made possible with the human genome project and other techniques that were made open access for researchers (Laird, 2010). The biomarkers which have shown much promise are DNA methylation-based biomarkers. Progress is now being made to explore if these biomarkers can help identify interventions to ameliorate the negative biological aspects of ageing. By using these biomarkers one can explore if the biological age is more or less than the chronological age. This then leads to exploring reasons for, and factors associated with, these differences and on to potential interventions.

Sociological Theories of Ageing

Successful Ageing Theory

This theory is based on studying those who live to and beyond the age of 100 years who also appear to live relatively free of chronic conditions and maintain their independence for much longer. It is postulated that this group have particularly good anti-inflammatory mechanisms that counterbalance the chronic low-grade inflammation associated with ageing. This balance influences whether ageing follows an accelerated, normal or decelerated pathway (Borras et al., 2020). There is a movement to describe the concept of healthy ageing and to identify the factors which contribute to successful ageing so that appropriate interventions can be developed. This contrasts with the previous focus on the negative aspects associated with ageing (Bowling and Dieppe, 2005). This focus on capacity rather than disease is also supported by WHO (World Report on Ageing and Health, 2015).

The Determinants of Well-Being and Health Theory

The determinants of well-being and health is another explanatory theory for how we age. This is popularly referred to as the social determinants of health (Figure 1.1) and WHO (2022) endorses this approach to understanding how our well-being and health is impacted by these factors.

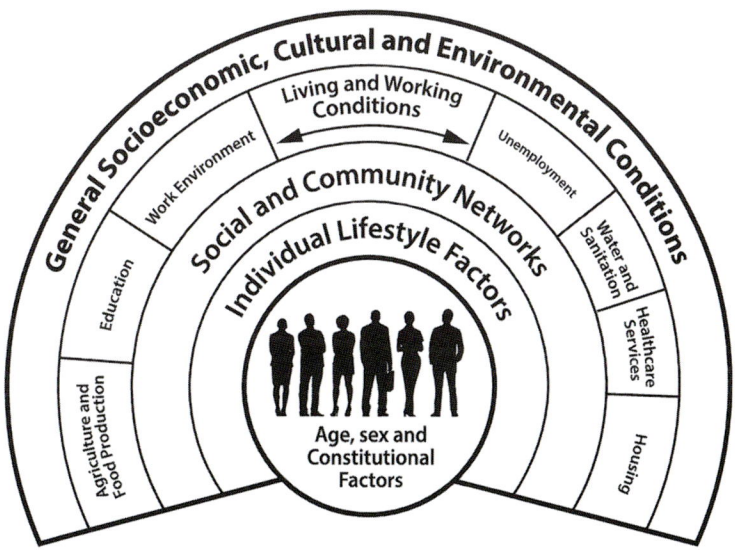

Figure 1.1 Social determinants of health.

Source: Dahlgren and Whitehead, 1991. Used with permission from the Institute for Futures Studies, Stockholm, Sweden.

Social determinants of health start from the moment a person is conceived and these can affect people into old age. For example, maternal well-being can influence the risk of developing non-communicable diseases in later life (Scher, 2013). The Helsinki birth cohort study also suggests that early childhood events contribute to the development of frailty in old age (Haapanen et al., 2018). Lifestyle choices, including dietary habits (Willett et al., 1999), alcohol consumption (van den Brandt and Brandts, 2020) and physical activity (Daskalopoulou et al., 2017), affect healthy ageing and life expectancy. An unhealthy environment can impact ageing negatively (Schmidt, 2019). For example, pollution can contribute to the development of frailty and sarcopenia in older people (de Amorim et al., 2019) and cognitive impairment (Lo et al., 2019). Figure 1.1 demonstrates how the many determinants can affect an individual.

Psychological Theories of Ageing

Stage Theories of Human Development

Human development and learning is lifelong, with previous experience influencing a person's well-being and health which can have positive benefits in old age. We know that even in later life, people can learn to change their lifestyle to impact positively on their well-being and health, which we will now explore (Hasworth and Cannon, 2015; Hearn et al., 2012; Latorre, 2015).

Cognitive Theories

The speed at which information is processed, abstract reasoning and solving problems in new situations declines with age while knowledge and skills attained tend to remain stable and can even get better (Horn and Cattell, 1967; Li, 2004). The brain has some reserve to deal with psychological and physical challenges on top of the usual day to day functions it must perform. This reserve reduces with getting older, but the speed at which it declines is impacted by the educational level of the individual and/or the degree to which the brain is stimulated by engaging in a variety of activities. It is therefore possible to influence this through a life course approach and then again in later life through some focussed support and training (Willis et al., 2009).

Emotional Theory

Our emotions and emotional experiences affect our physical and mental well-being throughout life (Charles and Carstensen, 2010). Several studies have suggested that older people prefer positive over negative information (Zarit, 2009; Reed, 2014). There also appears to be a deliberate attempt by older people to control and manage reactions to negative emotional experiences. The prefrontal area of the brain regulates this and conditions that damage this region affect this ability, for example traumatic brain injury, Alzheimer's disease, frontotemporal dementia or Parkinson's disease (Kryla-Lighthall and Mather, 2009; Carstensen et al., 2003).

Behavioural Theory

In this theory older people prioritise their life goals and activities as their physical and cognitive functional abilities decline. They also review their social network as they lose family and friends. Those who do this well tend to age successfully while those who struggle to come to terms with irreversible loss of function and how to adapt can find life difficult to cope with (Baltes and Baltes, 1990).

Physiology of Ageing

Ageing is a progressive process associated with an increased risk of developing chronic conditions, disability and death. The ageing of the organs in the human body occurs at different rates. Differences in lifespan can be explained by genetics in up to 25% of people with the determinants of well-being and health accounting for most of the rest (Passarino et al., 2016).

Homeostasis Changes

Older age is associated with changes in circadian rhythms, with body temperature, levels of hormones and sleep being affected. The secretion of some hormones such as gonadotropins, growth hormone, thyrotropin, melatonin and adrenocorticotropic hormone are impaired (Veldhuis, 1997; Van Cauter et al., 1996). There appears to be reduced variability in blood pressure, heart rate and stress response. This is described as loss of complexity (Lipsitz and Goldberger, 1992). Ageing is associated with a progressive reduction in physiological reserves to withstand stress resulting in an increased risk of illness. This was referred to as homeostenosis (Cowdry, 1942), but the concept of frailty is more commonly used now to explain this (see Chapter 3: Frailty).

Haematological Changes

In the haematopoietic system, enough capability is maintained throughout the life course, with normal red cell lifespan, iron turnover and blood volume, but the bone marrow mass is reduced with age. In old age, there are delayed responses to blood loss and hypoxia. While the total white cell numbers remain the same, the functioning of the several types of white cells declines increasing the risk of infection. Platelet numbers remain the same and there is an increased prothrombotic state in older adults (Yamamoto et al., 2005).

The changes which take place in the immune system are referred to as immunosenescence. These changes result in an increased risk of infections, inflammation, autoimmune diseases and neoplasms (Gustafson et al., 2020). Some of these changes include chronic low-grade inflammation usually associated with elevated inflammation markers (Franceschi et al., 2018), cell division arrest and resistance to cell death (Kirkland and Tchkonia, 2017). In addition to the impaired immune response in older adults, the following factors have been postulated to increase the risk of infections in older adults: the presence of multiple chronic conditions, impaired response to vaccines, impaired cough reflex, malnutrition and impaired mucosal barriers (Gavazzi and Krause, 2002). Pyrexia may be absent in up to 30% of older adults with infections (Norman, 2000). They tend to present with weakness, loss of appetite, falls and delirium and may not have the classical symptoms described in the textbooks for a younger adult population. Autoantibody production rises with age leading to an increased risk of autoimmune conditions. Just like in infections, older adults with autoimmune conditions, such as systemic lupus erythematosus, rheumatoid arthritis and Sjogren's syndrome, can present differently from younger adults. They can present with weight loss, muscle pain and cognitive impairment (Ramos-Casals et al., 2004).

Neurological Changes

In the central nervous system of older adults, there is often cerebral atrophy with the frontal and temporal lobes affected the most. More white than grey matter is lost and cerebral blood flow is also reduced (Driscoll et al., 2009; Salat et al., 1999). Executive function is vital in maintaining ADLs. This declines with ageing, especially after the age of 70 years (Harada et al., 2013). Concentration and multi-tasking also declines with ageing. This explains why older adults may be at an increased risk of falls, for example if their attention is on more than one task at a time (Smith et al., 2016; Yang et al., 2013).

Cardiovascular Changes

Changes in the cardiovascular system include reduced elastin, increased calcium deposits, accumulation of atherosclerosis, stiffness, increased systolic hypertension (this can fall in final years) and pulse wave velocity (Woodford, 2022). Heart failure occurs when the body's metabolic demands outweigh the capacity of the heart to pump at the required rate which is commonly caused due to the above changes, alongside reducing diastolic relaxation, and a potentially enlarged left ventricle (Woodford, 2022). The average age of diagnosis for heart failure is 77 years (Conrad et al., 2018).

Respiratory Changes

In the respiratory system of older adults, age associated changes increase the risk of hypoxia and pneumonia, for example there is a decreased surface area for gas exchange (Janssens, 2005). Ventilation perfusion mismatch contributes to a reduction in arterial PaO_2 with ageing and is more marked in women and those in the supine position (Hardie et al., 2002). There are no changes in $PaCO_2$ with ageing (Hardie, 2004). Abdominal muscles contribute more to chest wall expansion in older adults because the diaphragm is less efficient (Woodford, 2022). The ability to clear secretions is impaired with ageing (Ho et al., 2001).

Gastrointestinal Changes

In the gastrointestinal system about 50% of older adults will have a dry mouth, a condition that is exacerbated by some of the medications they are prescribed (Smith et al., 2013; Nagler and Hershkovich, 2005). There are also changes in the oesophageal muscle contractions in older adults which, coupled with tongue movement impairment, increases the risk of aspiration (Frederick et al., 1996; Iyota et al., 2020). The risk of gastritis increases in older adults because of reduced synthesis of prostaglandins and bicarbonate coupled with delayed emptying of the stomach (Guslandi et al., 1999). Intestinal neurons are reduced contributing to an increased incidence of older adults unable to feel pain due to ulcers (Hall et al., 2005; Hilton et al., 2001) and the perception of pain with bowel perforation, distention or ischaemia is impaired which can delay timely diagnosis (Lagier et al., 1999). Motility in the large intestine is reduced with about 25% of older adults developing constipation (Dunn-Walters et al., 2004). Older adult women have a reduced anal sphincter tone, which could account for the increased risk of faecal incontinence seen (Gundling et al., 2010). Liver function is relatively well preserved except for about a third of older adults with a reduced drug clearance due to reductions in cytochrome P450 (McLachlan and Pont, 2012).

Renal Changes

The changes in the renal system in older people include a smaller renal mass with an increase in fat and fibrosis, sclerosis of cortical nephrons, reduction in renal blood flow and creatinine clearance, defective sodium and potassium excretion and conservation and reduction in concentrating and diluting capacity. This makes the older adult kidney more sensitive to injuries which it will take longer to recover from (Taffet, 2003).

Genitourinary Changes

The changes in the genitourinary system increase the risk of dyspareunia, erectile dysfunction, urinary tract infection and urinary incontinence. Urinary incontinence is more common in older adult women up until the age of 80 years when there are no differences between men and women. The increased risk of urinary incontinence is due to reduction in detrusor muscle contractility, bladder capacity, flow rate and the ability to withhold voiding (Elbadawi et al., 1998). The length of the urethra and its closure pressure is reduced because of the lack of oestrogen in older adult women. This increases the risk of infection (Dubeau, 2006). The vagina loses elasticity, and becomes atrophic and dry. It becomes less acidic, allowing colonisation by enteric microflora. In men the prostate gland enlarges with ageing.

Musculoskeletal Changes

In the musculoskeletal system, muscle mass and strength reduce with ageing resulting in sarcopenia with the legs being more affected than the arms. Recovery after injury is also impaired (Snijders et al., 2014). There is a gradual reduction in bone mass in older adults which is more marked in women after the menopause. Following a fracture, healing is also impaired (Chan and Duque, 2002; Meyer, 2006).

Dermatological Changes

The skin atrophies with ageing and there is a reduction in its elasticity. It becomes thinner and more prone to injury. Thermoregulation is impaired increasing the risk of older adults being unable to cope with elevated temperatures and being unable to respond appropriately to low temperatures (Tan et al., 2020).

Vision, Hearing, Taste and Smell Changes

The most common eye changes in older adults are refractive errors and cataracts, both of which can be treated successfully (Swenor et al., 2020). Changes in the ear

CHAPTER 1 Theories and Physiology of Ageing

result in loss of hearing acuity, difficulty with speech discrimination and localising the sources of sound (Howarth and Shone, 2006). There is a gradual loss of taste and smell which can impact appetite and food intake in older adults (Boyce and Shone, 2006; Mojet et al., 2001).

Conclusion

The theories of ageing and physiology discussed in this chapter paint a clinical picture of ageing. It provides older people and those who care for them with a better understanding of how best to support and initiate appropriate interventions to address what matters to them (Akpan et al., 2018). It also implies that a preventive life course approach can be taken to mitigate the impacts of some of the irreversible declines that will occur. Not all adults will experience all the changes associated with ageing, but most will live through a combination of two or more, each being different for each individual. This, therefore, goes some way to begin to explain the wide variation of the lived experience of this important patient group.

> ### Questions
>
> 1. Consider this chapter's content and apply what you have learnt to a recent patient or family member.
> 2. How does the information reframe your assessment?
> 3. Which of the theories described can you identify with your patient?

References

Akpan A, et al. (2018). Standard set of health outcome measures for older persons. *BMC Geriatrics*, 18(1): 36.

Baltes PB, Baltes MM (1990). Psychological perspectives on successful aging: the model of selective optimization with compensation. In *Successful Aging: Perspectives from the behavioral sciences*, Baltes PB and Baltes MM (eds.). Cambridge, UK: Cambridge University Press: 1–34.

Borras C, et al. (2020). Centenarians: an excellent example of resilience for successful ageing. *Mechanisms of Ageing and Development*, 186: 111199.

Bowling A, Dieppe P (2005). What is successful ageing and who should define it? *British Medical Journal*, 331(7531): 1548–1551.

Boyce JM, Shone GR (2006). Effects of ageing on smell and taste. *Postgraduate Medical Journal*, 82(966): 239–241.

Carstensen L, Fung H, Charles S (2003). Socioemotional selectivity theory and the regulation of emotion in the second half of life. *Motivation and Emotion*, 27(2): 103–123.

Chan GK, Duque G (2002). Age-related bone loss: old bone, new facts. *Gerontology*, 48(2): 62–71.

Charles ST, Carstensen LL (2010). Social and emotional aging. *Annual Review of Psychology*, 61: 383–409.

Chaudhary MR, et al. (2023). Aging, oxidative stress and degenerative diseases: mechanisms, complications and emerging therapeutic strategies. *Biogerontology*, 24: 609–662.

Conrad N, et al. (2018). Temporal trends and patterns in mortality after incident heart failure: a longitudinal analysis of 86 000 individuals. *JAMA Cardiology*, 4(11): 1102–1111.

References

Cowdry EV (1942). *Problems of Ageing: Biological and medical aspects* (2nd edition). Baltimore: Williams & Wilkins.

Dahlgren G, Whitehead M (1991). *Policies and Strategies to Promote Social Equity in Health*. Stockholm: Institute for Futures Studies.

Daskalopoulou C, et al. (2017). Physical activity and healthy ageing: a systematic review and meta-analysis of longitudinal cohort studies. *Ageing Research Reviews*, 38: 6–17.

de Amorim JSC, et al. (2019). Factors associated with the prevalence of sarcopenia and frailty syndrome in elderly university workers. *Archives of Gerontology and Geriatrics*, 82: 172–178.

Driscoll I, et al. (2009). Longitudinal pattern of regional brain volume change differentiates normal aging from MCI. *Neurology*, 72(22): 1906–1913.

Dubeau CE (2006). The aging lower urinary tract. *Journal of Urology*, 175(3 Pt 2): S11–S15.

Dunn-Walters DK, Howard WA, Bible JM (2004). The ageing gut. *Mechanism of Ageing and Development*, 125(12): 851–85.

Elbadawi A, Diokno AC, Millard RJ (1998). The aging bladder: morphology and urodynamics. *World Journal of Urology*, 16 (Suppl 1): S10–34.

Franceschi C, et al. (2018). Inflammaging: a new immune-metabolic viewpoint for age-related diseases. *Nature Reviews Endocrinology*, 14(10): 576–590.

Frederick MG, et al. (1996). Functional abnormalities of the pharynx: a prospective analysis of radiographic abnormalities relative to age and symptoms. *American Journal of Roentgenology*, 166(2): 353–357.

Gavazzi G, Krause KH (2002). Ageing and infection. *The Lancet Infectious Diseases*, 2(11): 659–666.

Gundling F, et al. (2010). Influence of gender and age on anorectal function: normal values from anorectal manometry in a large caucasian population. *Digestion*, 81(4): 207–213.

Guslandi M, Pellegrini A, Sorghi M (1999). Gastric mucosal defences in the elderly. *Gerontology*, 45(4): 206–208.

Gustafson CE, et al. (2020). Influence of immune aging on vaccine responses. *Journal of Allergy and Clinical Immunology*, 145(5): 1309–1321.

Haapanen MJ et al. (2018). Early life determinants of frailty in old age: the Helsinki Birth Cohort Study. *Age and Ageing*, 47(4): 569–575.

Hall KE, et al. (2005). American gastroenterological association future trends committee report: effects of aging of the population on gastroenterology practice, education, and research. *Gastroenterology*, 129(4): 1305–1338.

Harada CN, Natelson Love MC, Triebel KL (2013). Normal cognitive aging. *Clinics in Geriatric Medicine*, 29(4): 737–752.

Hardie JA, Mørkve O, Ellingsen I (2002). Effect of body position on arterial oxygen tension in the elderly. *Respiration*, 69(2): 123–128.

Hardie JA, et al. (2004). Reference values for arterial blood gases in the elderly. *Chest*, 125(6): 2053–2060.

Harman D (1956). Aging: a theory based on free radical and radiation chemistry. *Journal of Gerontology*, 11(3): 298–300.

Harman D (1978). Free radical theory of aging: nutritional implications. *Age*, 1: 145–152.

Hasworth S, Cannon M (2015). Social theories of aging. *Disease-a-Month*, 61(11): 475–479.

Hearn S, et al. (2012). Between integrity and despair: toward construct validation of Erikson's eighth stage. *The Journal of Adult Development*, 19(1): 1–20.

Hilton D, et al. (2001). Absence of abdominal pain in older persons with endoscopic ulcers: a prospective study. *American Journal of Gastroenterology*, 96(2): 380–384.

Ho JC, et al. (2001). The effect of aging on nasal mucociliary clearance, beat frequency, and ultrastructure of respiratory cilia. *American Journal of Respiratory and Critical Care Medicine*, 163(4): 983–988.

CHAPTER 1 Theories and Physiology of Ageing

Horn JL, Cattell RB (1967). Age differences in fluid and crystallized intelligence. *Acta Psychologica*, 26(2): 107–129.

Horvath S, Raj K (2018). DNA methylation-based biomarkers and the epigenetic clock theory of ageing. *Nature Reviews Genetics*, 19(6): 371–384.

Howarth A, Shone GR (2006). Ageing and the auditory system. *Postgraduate Medical Journal*, 82(965): 166–171.

Iyota K, et al. (2020). Cross-sectional study of age-related changes in oral function in healthy Japanese individuals. *International Journal of Environmental Research and Public Health*, 17(4): 1376.

Janssens JP (2005). Aging of the respiratory system: impact on pulmonary function tests and adaptation to exertion. *Clinics in Chest Medicine*, 26(3): 469–484.

Kirkland JL, Tchkonia T (2017). Cellular senescence: a translational perspective. *EBioMedicine*, 21: 21–28.

Kryla-Lighthall N, Mather M (2009). The role of cognitive control in older adults' emotional well-being. In *Handbook of Theories of Aging* (2nd edition). New York: Springer: 323–344.

Lagier E, et al. (1999). Influence of age on rectal tone and sensitivity to distension in healthy subjects. *Neurogastroenterology and Motility*, 11(2): 101–107.

Laird PW (2010). Principles and challenges of genome-wide DNA methylation analysis. *Nature Reviews Genetics*, 11: 191–203.

Latorre JM, et al. (2015). Life review based on remembering specific positive events in active aging. *Journal of Aging and Health*, 27(1): 140–157.

Li S-C, et al. (2004). Transformations in the couplings among intellectual abilities and constituent cognitive processes across the life span. *Psychological Science*, 15(3): 155–163.

Lipsitz LA, Goldberger AL (1992). Loss of 'complexity' and aging. Potential applications of fractals and chaos theory to senescence. *Journal of the American Medical Association*, 267(13): 1806–1809.

Lipsky MS, King M (2015). Biological theories of aging. *Disease-a-Month*, 61(11): 460–466.

Lo YC, et al. (2019). Air pollution exposure and cognitive function in Taiwanese older adults: a repeated measurement study. *Int J Environ Res Public Health*, 16(16): 2976.

McLachlan AJ, Pont LG (2012). Drug metabolism in older people – a key consideration in achieving optimal outcomes with medicines. *The Journals of Gerontology: Series A*, 67A(2): 175–180.

Meyer RA Jr, et al. (2006). Young, adult, and old rats have similar changes in mRNA expression of many skeletal genes after fracture despite delayed healing with age. *Journal of Orthopaedic Research*, 24(10): 1933–1944.

Mojet J, Christ-Hazelhof E, Heidema J (2001). Taste perception with age: generic or specific losses in threshold sensitivity to the five basic tastes? *Chemical Senses*, 26(7): 845–860.

Nagler RM, Hershkovich O (2005). Age-related changes in unstimulated salivary function and composition and its relations to medications and oral sensorial complaints. *Aging Clinical and Experimental Research*, 17(5): 358–366.

Norman DC (2000). Fever in the elderly. *Clinical Infectious Diseases*, 31(1): 148–151.

Passarino G, De Rango F, Montesanto A (2016). Human longevity: genetics or lifestyle? It takes two to tango. *Immunity and Ageing*, 13(1): 12.

Pomatto LCD, et al. (2018). Aging attenuates redox adaptive homeostasis and proteostasis in female mice exposed to traffic-derived nanoparticles ('vehicular smog'). *Free Radical Biology and Medicine*, 121: 86–97.

Ramos-Casals M, et al. (2004). Systemic autoimmune diseases in elderly patients: atypical presentation and association with neoplasia. *Autoimmunity Reviews*, 3(5): 376–382.

Reed AE, Chan L, Mikels JA (2014). Meta-analysis of the age-related positivity effect: age differences in preferences for positive over negative information. *Psychology and Aging*, 29(1): 1–15

References

Salat DH, Kaye JA, Janowsky JS (1999). Prefrontal gray and white matter volumes in healthy aging and Alzheimer disease. *Archives of Neurology*, 56(3): 338–444.

Scher M (2013). Normal and abnormal cerebrovascular development: gene–environment interactions during early life with later life consequences. *Handbook of Clinical Neurology*, 112: 1021–1042.

Schmidt CW (2019). Environmental factors in successful aging: the potential impact of air pollution. *Environmental Health Perspectives*, 127:10.

Smith CH, et al. (2013). Effect of aging on stimulated salivary flow in adults. *Journal of the American Geriatrics Society*, 61(5): 805–808.

Smith E, Cusack T, Blake C (2016). The effect of a dual task on gait speed in community dwelling older adults: a systematic review and meta-analysis. *Gait and Posture*, 44: 250–258.

Snijders T, et al. (2014). The skeletal muscle satellite cell response to a single bout of resistance-type exercise is delayed with aging in men. *Age (Dordr) Journal*, 36(4): 9699.

Speakman JR, Selman C (2011). The free-radical damage theory: accumulating evidence against a simple link of oxidative stress to ageing and lifespan. *Bioessays*, 33(4): 255–259.

Stadtman ER (1992). Protein oxidation and aging. *Science*, 257(5074): 1220–1224.

Swenor BK, et al. (2020). Aging with vision loss: a framework for assessing the impact of visual impairment on older adults. *The Gerontologist*, 60(6): 989–995.

Taffet GE (2003). Physiology of aging. In *Geriatric Medicine: An evidence-based approach* (4th edition), Cassel C (ed.). New York: Springer: 27–35.

Tan CCS, Chin LKK, Low ICC (2020). Thermoregulation in the aging population and practical strategies to overcome a warmer tomorrow. *Proteomics*, 20(5–6): e1800468.

Van Cauter E, Leproult R, Kupfer DJ (1996). Effects of gender and age on the levels and circadian rhythmicity of plasma cortisol. *Journal of Clinical Endocrinology and Metabolism*, 81(7): 2468–2473.

van den Brandt PA, Brandts L (2020). Alcohol consumption in later life and reaching longevity: the Netherlands Cohort Study. *Age and Ageing*, 49(3): 395–402.

Varela-López A, et al. (2023). Dietary antioxidants and lifespan: relevance of environmental conditions, diet, and genotype of experimental models. *Experimental Gerontology*, 178: 112221.

Veldhuis JD (1997). Altered pulsatile and coordinate secretion of pituitary hormones in aging: evidence of feedback disruption. *Aging (Milano)*, 9(4 Suppl): 19–20.

Willett WC, Dietz WH, Colditz GA (1999). Guidelines for healthy weight. *New England Journal of Medicine*, 341(6): 427–434.

Willis SL, Schaie KW, Martin M (2009). Cognitive plasticity. In *Handbook of Theories of Aging* (2nd edition), Bengston VL et al. (eds.). New York: Springer; 2009: 295–322.

Woodford HJ (2022). *Essential geriatrics. Ageing* (4th edition). Oxon: CRC Press.

World Health Organization (2015). World report on ageing and health. Available at: https://apps.who.int/iris/bitstream/handle/10665/186463/9?sequence=1 [accessed 2nd May 2024].

World Health Organization (2022). Social determinants of health. Available at: https://www.who.int/health-topics/social-determinants-of-health#tab=tab_1 [accessed 2nd May 2024].

Yamamoto K, et al. (2005). Aging and plasminogen activator inhibitor-1 (PAI-1) regulation: implication in the pathogenesis of thrombotic disorders in the elderly. *Cardiovascular Research*, 66(2): 276–285.

Yang AC, et al. (2013). Complexity of spontaneous BOLD activity in default mode network is correlated with cognitive function in normal male elderly: a multiscale entropy analysis. *Neurobiology of Aging*, 34(2): 428–438.

Zarit SH (2009). A good old age: theories of mental health and aging. In *Handbook of Theories of Aging* (2nd edition), Bengston VL et al. (eds.). New York: Springer: 675–691.

Chapter 2

Person-Centred Communication

Gemma Howlett

> **Learning Points**
>
> By the end of this chapter, you will:
> - Understand what person-centred communication is
> - Have learnt about some barriers to person-centred communication
> - Be able to recognise unconscious bias and stereotypes
> - Have the tools to move towards more person-centred communication.

Please note the focus of this chapter is communication with the older person, therefore the case study will be framed differently from those in the other chapters. The clinical elements will have less of a focus and instead the chapter will look at specific areas of communication that we must consider in our treatment of older people.

> **Case Study**
>
> You are responding on a double crewed ambulance to reports of a 74-year-old man called John who has fallen in the garden and has badly hurt his knee; he is in a lot of pain and is unable to move. The call was made around three hours prior to your arrival time.
>
> The patient fell while jumping over a section of the garden where he had just planted some bulbs and did not want to stand on them. He landed awkwardly and thinks he twisted his leg which caused the fall to the ground. John thinks he heard a crack as he fell and is stating that the pain is the worst pain he has ever felt. He took some paracetamol around an hour before you arrived on scene, but it has not had any effect. In the garden with the patient is a woman and a man around the same age as John.

CHAPTER 2 Person-Centred Communication

Introduction

Healthcare communication is an interdependent process: each involved party is reliant on the other for information (Pagano, 2015). The clinician needs information from the patient or a family member on a variety of often complex subjects such as presenting complaint, family history, medical history and social history to start to develop a working diagnosis and treatment plan with the patient (Pagano, 2015). Patients in turn need information from healthcare providers to understand what is happening and make their own decisions around their care (Pagano, 2015). It seems obvious to say that good communication is essential for good patient care. However, it is clear from an abundance of evidence and serious incidents that in the NHS and other patient and clinical settings it regularly goes wrong with significant consequences (Campbell et al., 2018; GMC, 2019).

What is Person-Centred Communication?

Person-centred care is the approach that is advocated for in all UK healthcare systems. It is a shared decision-making process between clinician and patient which is based on best medical evidence and the person's individual preferences, beliefs and values (NICE, 2021). There has been a shift away from paternalistic practices of physician led and directed care. Instead there is now a focus on working in partnership with our patients to ensure they are included and also empowered to determine and influence their treatment choices. Evidence suggests that when the patient is actively involved in their own care they better understand what is being proposed and are more likely to better manage their illness or symptoms, and to engage with further support (Naughton, 2018). Involvement in their own care can also significantly reduce patient stress and anxiety, and lead to a safer and more satisfying care experience (Naughton, 2018). To enable this method of care we need to move to a person-centred communication strategy. It is not a simple case of outlining a list of questions under specific headings that we see commonly in some of the communication literature. If it were as simplistic as a unifocal 'how to list' then we could assume that more people would be communicating this way with their patients, but the evidence suggests that this is not the case.

Communication Breakdowns

Storlie (2015) found in their research around communication with older people that there are five main causal factors commonly seen when looking at communication breakdowns, poor practice and clinical errors which were directly attributed to poor communication. These are:

- Ageist attitudes and language
- A lack of provider commitment to person-centred service delivery and patient care
- Inappropriate use of professional jargon by the provider
- Underdeveloped communication skills of the provider
- Impediments to effective communication stemming from cultural differences and from age-related physical, social and psychological changes in the older adult.

The list provides five areas of focus that will be explored individually throughout the rest of this chapter, using the case study to examine potential pitfalls, and importantly solutions and strategies to utilise when communicating with our older patients.

Ageism

We all have a variety of unconscious or implicit biases, which are beliefs we have about groups of people in relation to, for example, their race, gender, sexual orientation, disability, age or socioeconomic group (Wilson et al., 2021). These biases are created through factors such as our education, upbringing, influence of our family and friends, experiences and exposures which form the lens through which we see the world and the people in it (Wilson et al., 2021).

Ageist attitudes and tropes are present in everyday language, in the media and press, social media, marketing, film and television. Older adults are commonly shown through a lens of decline and diminishing value in society, often emphasising the 'burden' that older people place on society and families (Milner et al., 2012). These daily images reinforce stereotypes, enforce prejudice and misconceptions, and underpin discriminatory behaviour (Centre for Ageing Better, 2021). The pervasive societal stereotype around older adults is that they are less competent than younger people (Wilson et al., 2021). Older people are commonly portrayed as frail, vulnerable and dependent (Centre for Ageing Better, 2021). It has been difficult to shift this attitude and it has significant effects on care and treatment received in all facets of life for older people.

Ageist stereotypes and biases permeate across society. Judi Dench famously brought up these stereotypes and biases which are present within the paramedic profession. In the film *Nothing Like a Dame* she describes an encounter with a paramedic following a sting on her bottom from a hornet. The paramedic opened the interaction with 'And what is our name?' with the second question being 'And do we have a carer?' Judi openly expresses her anger about the biases and stereotypical attitudes and assumptions surrounding older people.

There is also a need to consider the intersectionality issues of bias and stereotyping. Pedersen and Nielsen (2019) when considering gender bias identified that women and men (or those who identify as such) are often stereotyped according to the traits that they are assumed to possess, which leads in many instances to unequal treatment based solely on gender. Social identity theory states that demographic characteristics such as race or gender shape socialisation experiences which influence and affect identity formation, attitude, belief and perceptions (Pedersen and Nielsen, 2019). When considering these intersects, an older woman will face both gender stereotyping and discrimination as well as stereotyping and bias surrounding her age. An older black woman may face biases and discrimination based on her race in addition to her gender and age. We all need to be aware of this as clinicians, and think about the stereotypes and biases that we take into patient encounters often without thinking. It will have very real consequences and significantly influence how we communicate with our patients if we do not acknowledge these factors and start to try and address them.

Now let us revisit John, our patient in the case study. What assumptions did you make about him when you read about the incident in the garden?

CHAPTER 2   Person-Centred Communication

Your brain would have automatically started filling in the gaps and painting the picture of that encounter; it would have started placing the various people in the scenario into categories, to make sense of the situation. The brain does not like an incomplete story. The snippets of information that you get on your way to a patient if responding for the ambulance service, or before a consultation, allow space for assumptions. What might you have assumed about John? Did you consider that John still worked? He was a lawyer before semi-retirement and now acts as a consultant for several law firms throughout the country. He is well renowned and respected in his field.

Would this have been the first thing that came into your mind do you think when you read that you were responding to an older male patient who had fallen in his garden?

Honest reflection and consideration of this helps to understand our stereotypes and biases. It is only when we start acknowledging these, reflecting on the factors that contribute to these stereotypes, that we can start to address them. We also need to consider the other people in the patient encounter. It is often as important in patient-centred communication that you build a relationship with those who are closest to the patient and work with them, as well as the patient, to arrive at a co-constructed treatment plan.

How may you have greeted the woman in the case study? Women are often called 'love' or 'dear' or 'flower' (insert your own local term for an older woman); we will explore some of the reasons for this later in the chapter. Men often command more respect: they will commonly be greeted as 'sir' or 'boss' (again, insert your own standard local greeting) initially. What assumptions would you have made about her? Who is she to John? Many of us would assume she is his wife, based on age and the fact that she is in the garden with him. She is in fact his sister Wendy who has lived with him for several years. The other man in the scenario – who is he? He is John's husband, Steve; he came home from work when John and Wendy called to say that John had fallen and was unable to get up. Granted you were not given much information to be able to determine this from the initial description, but this is the reality of frontline healthcare, these are the snippets, the quick pictures, the hasty views that you will have initially. What assumptions would you have made? How would you have asked who everyone was? It is unrealistic to expect you to know exactly who everyone is at the scene in relation to the patient, and indeed who the patient is or anything about them, and that is exactly the point: do not guess, do not assume – ask and learn.

Lack of Provider Commitment

It should go without saying that all people matter, irrespective of their age, race, sexual orientation, gender, religion or any other category they may be put into. Unfortunately for many people this is not their experience of healthcare. People want to be seen for who they are, they want to feel that they are valued, that their opinions and ideas about their care and their life matter to the healthcare clinician involved in their care and to have their undivided attention even if only for a few minutes (Storlie, 2015). Safe and trustful communication between healthcare providers and patients is essential for reducing healthcare injuries and negative experiences (Johnsson et al., 2018). At the heart of communication must be the patient: their values, their preferences, their expressed needs and their direct involvment in their own care (Johnsson et al., 2018). It must be considerate of the person's individuality, humanity, dignity, right to be recognised and their ability to bring their whole self to the situation (Hewitt-Taylor, 2015), irrespective of any protected characteristics or their socioeconomic status (which is not recognised in the equality act currently).

Jensen et al. (2021) in their work on person-centred care in the emergency department (ED), noted that the high-intensity workflow is characterised by a constant level of uncertainty and unpredictability around which patient will present next. This is the same for frontline clinicians in the paramedic profession and advanced clinical practitioners (ACPs) within the community and leads to a challenging environment in which it is difficult to conduct unhurried person-centred care conversations. It is, however, essential that we do include our patients in the decisions we help them to make, either with them as individuals or with the help of their family members. Involving our patients in their care and allowing them to inform and direct their treatment choices leads to a patient who has been supported and empowered by the healthcare system to subsequently become more engaged in their care plan thus improving outcomes in the long term (Jensen et al., 2021).

John is married to Steve and identifies as queer or gay. Studies looking at LGBTQIA+ experiences of healthcare have demonstrated that providers' biases can range from subtle covert behaviours, known as microaggressions, to blatant homophobia, biphobia and transphobic discrimination (Smith and Turell, 2019). John and Steve would have seen the portrayal of gay men during the AIDS epidemic; they will have been aware and out in society when Section 28 was in situ which prohibited the 'promotion' or discussion of homosexuality. This is all a part of their story and history. Much of healthcare policy and education centres around heteronormativity. As a result, LGBTQIA+ individuals are missed out from the outset. They frequently report discomfort in healthcare situations, and often feel the need to withhold information, change providers to avoid a provider knowing too much or following a negative experience, or they do not seek healthcare at all (Smith and Turell, 2019). A lack of inclusion and involvement in their own care has had lasting damaging effects on many members of the LGBTQIA+ community, as it will do for other marginalised groups and those who have felt excluded from their care, or have experienced poor communication during healthcare encounters. Healthcare practitioners must understand how important communication is and want to fully engage with it to avoid experiences such as these. Individuals must value its importance and see it as a priority in order to deliver person-centred care consistently and successfully.

Jargon

Research indicates that there is a mismatch between what the healthcare providers think they have communicated and what the patients hear and understand following healthcare contact (Miller et al., 2021). Providers generally think that they consistently speak in plain language to their patients, but clinicians routinely overestimate the patients' understanding of medical terminology or jargon (Miller et al., 2021). Jargon is one of the core barriers to effective communication. It is routinely used in patient interactions by clinicians and is overly complex, confusing and often in complete opposition to respectful person-centred communication (Stone et al., 2021). Jargon and complicated medical terminology should always be avoided. Where there is any doubt that your patient may not understand what is being said, active listening, clarifying questions and asking the patients to relay their understanding back are all tools that can aid understanding and foster a respectful professional relationship between you and your patient.

Underdeveloped Communication Skills

Good communication, with a clear and consistent focus on a person-centred approach, is not easy. It is something, irrespective of your length of service, grade or age, that needs to be practised, routinely reflected on and, as with other elements of care, implemented with a consistent view to best evidence and a commitment to maintaining and honing the skills required. An inability to build rapport, a lack of active listening strategies, a lack of openness and a lack of questions due to assumptions already being made and relied upon as fact will cause significant communication problems.

Storlie (2015) encourages clinicians, when reflecting on their communication with older adults, to consider the following contemplative questions:

- Is your communication with older adults mostly person-centred, is it generally effective, always respectful and do you think it is mutually satisfying? If so, why? What are you doing and/or not doing that is creating this experience for you and your older patient? List some of the areas where you feel that you have strengths, and identify any areas where you feel you need to make improvements.

- Identify someone who you believe communicates effectively and respectfully with older adults. What is it that the person does that enables them to have these effective person-centred conversations? List the major factors and imagine how you can start to build these techniques into your own communication.

Regular reflection on patient contacts with a focus on communication, as with other areas of practice, is an effective way of making improvements. It will help you develop your person-centred communication skills and enable you to help your older patients make the decision that is right for them.

Cultural Differences and Age-Related Changes

Barriers to true person-centred communication and care can include resources, policies and the structure of the organisation involved, workplace culture and values, individual clinician beliefs, values and priorities (Hewitt-Taylor, 2015). In addition to these barriers there are the physical and cognitive barriers that are often assumed to be present in the older adult based purely on the age of the patient and the biases surrounding them. You need to ascertain when you have met the patient whether there are any physical barriers or impediments that you need to be aware of. Do not assume there is a deficit in hearing and automatically talk very loudly to the patient.

It can be seen as patronising and disrespectful. If there is a deficit in hearing, sight or any other barrier to them communicating with you, then find out where possible how they like to communicate. What do they need? Would it be useful for instance to write things down for them? Or, if wearing personal protective equipment, would it help to remove your mask to enable lipreading?

Culture, or difference in culture, needs to be considered when trying to build a rapport with the patient and/or family. Culturally competent communication needs to be at the heart of person-centred communication. If we fail to acknowledge the patient's culture, celebrate their differences, and allow the unique elements of individuals to inform their care and the decisions that they make, then we are failing them. Brooks et al. (2018) state that culturally competent communication is the effective verbal and nonverbal interactions between a patient and healthcare provider where a mutual understanding and respect of each other's values, beliefs, preferences and culture is present, and the objective is to achieve a culturally sensitive care and treatment plan for the individual. It is unrealistic to expect you to know all there is about every culture and even if this were the case, there would still be a level of assumption present. It is not the case that everyone from a certain culture will wish to be treated the same. What instead needs to be a core focus is the absolute desire to learn with the patient and family, where appropriate and applicable, about each individual patient and the care they wish to receive.

Moving Towards Person-Centred Care

Throughout the literature there are many communication models proposed for use in healthcare. It is an often-overwhelming task searching through them all. Much of the literature on communication with older persons still maintains an increased focus on the 'deficits' of ageing, concentrating on frailty, loss of sight, hearing and so on, and overcoming these deficits (Eliassen, 2015). This not only replicates stereotypical tropes of ageing but firmly establishes a power dynamic between healthcare provider and patient, framing all patients as vulnerable and in need of extra care (Eliassen, 2015). However, the older population is increasingly diverse. There is a growing majority of adults moving into their 60s still physically and mentally able, active and socially engaged, with many choosing or having to work beyond standard retirement age (Eliassen, 2015). It is important that you move away from assumptions and stereotypes, starting your dialogue with the patient respectfully and openly, in order to get to their truth and their needs. Simple strategies include making sure you get down to the patient's level if they are sitting or lying down as it is intimidating to be towered over. Shake hands (if this is appropriate) and use a kind approach. Ensure you ask how they would like to be addressed, as the wrong greeting can cause an instant barrier. Use open body language, active and attentive listening, minimise distractions around the patient and if you are working with a colleague, involve the patient in your discussions with them. Try and arrange additional support for those who may have difficulties with partaking in shared decision making, particularly if there is not a family member, friend or carer available to help or, importantly, if the patient does not want them involved (NICE, 2021).

Person-centred care must focus on getting to know the person, including their history, values, beliefs, priorities, understanding of the current situation, responsibilities,

CHAPTER 2 Person-Centred Communication

preferences, future aspirations and how they are making sense of – or how they understand – what is happening and what the potential plans are (Hewitt-Taylor, 2015). You effectively need to enter your patient's world, to try and understand how they see things. It does not mean that you must agree with their perceptions or ideas or adopt them as your own while with them, but instead you should be able to view matters through the eyes of the person you are treating, understanding and appreciating how these factors and their individuality shapes and influences their reality and choices (Hewitt-Taylor, 2015). This respect for self-determination of the patient does not mean that you should withdraw totally from the decision-making process. The patient needs your help; they need your guidance and expertise as well as your understanding of the evidence and the likely consequences of the choices they are considering. However, what this conversation cannot be is coercive or intentionally leading (Hewitt-Taylor, 2015). NICE (2021) stipulate clearly that when you are giving information to the patient then you must use high-quality evidence and not lead the patient incorrectly. These conversations, preferences, fears, values and cultural influences need to be documented so that the shared decision can be evidenced and used by ongoing clinicians.

To offer this care and build the required partnership, the healthcare clinician must continually develop their communication and observation skills, reflecting on both positive and negative experiences. It is not something that many people are going to be instantly good at. It is important that you not only focus on medical knowledge and technical clinical skills but also develop cognitive and emotional intelligence skills. Ongoing reflection and development of these skills is important.

The proposed communication model outlined in Table 2.1 merges and adapts the work of Naughton (2018) and Silverman (2016) and offers some guidance on the core components of the person-centred communication strategy.

Table 2.1 A person-centred communication strategy.

Objective	Healthcare Clinician	Communication Skills
Foster the relationship	Build a rapport with patient and family Appear open Demonstrate respect Demonstrate care and commitment Acknowledge the patient's feelings and emotions	Warm respectful greeting Unbiased approach Maintain eye contact Show interest, be attentive Listen actively Express empathy
Gather information	Determine the purpose of current patient encounter Discover primary complaint Explore patient expectations Get to know patient What matters to them	Open-ended questions Allow patient the time to complete their responses Do not rush Clarify and summarise regularly Explore the impact of illness on patient

Objective	Healthcare Clinician	Communication Skills
Provide the correct amount and type of information	Assessing where the patient is starting from – what do they know already? Regularly check understanding to ensure the patient is with you at each step Aid accurate recall	Check understanding at each stage Can the patient repeat what has been said? Teach back method (NICE, 2021): patient to 'teach back' what has been discussed, deeper than 'do you understand?'
Achieve a shared understanding	Relating explanations to patient's perspectives Providing opportunities to contribute Picking up cues Eliciting reactions and feelings	Check your own understanding of the patient's perspective Check understanding at each stage Explore any anxiety around treatment Validate patient's feelings Open and empathetic approach
Shared decision making	Sharing thinking Involving the patient Exploring options Ascertaining level of involvement patient wishes Negotiating mutually acceptable plan	Explore the patient's preferences Identify and explore any barriers to treatment Check understanding at each stage Identify any barriers to potential self-management Ensure these are relayed to next stage care clinicians

Communication with Other Healthcare Providers

As with our patient interactions, good communication is essential when we are relaying information to, or liaising with, other professionals to establish a care plan and care strategy for our patients. Both mechanisms involve a complex mix of formal and informal communication which is both verbal and written. Failures in communication during handover are a major cause of critical incidents (Eggins et al., 2016). Patient-centred communication and care, as discussed and rationalised in detail within this chapter, must be at the heart of all interactions with our patients, and this includes handover. Evidence suggests that patients should also be central and involved in the handover process. Having the patient central in the handover process emphasises shared patient and clinician decision making, it demands transparency and honesty around the patient's care and helps continue or further develop rapport with the patient (Eggins et al., 2016). Evidence suggests that this involvement results in fewer misunderstandings, greater compliance with treatment and therefore fewer

CHAPTER 2 Person-Centred Communication

healthcare contacts (Eggins et al., 2016). Including the patient necessitates that you explain all elements appropriately and clearly. It dictates that you would not be able to use jargon and incorrectly assume that another healthcare provider knows and understands what you are saying. It ensures that both the patient and the receiving clinician is fully aware of what has been done and what is being proposed.

Conclusion

Person-centred communication is not simple or easy; however, it is the best way to care for our patients. Person-centred care encourages us to look beyond the illness or injury that the patient presents with, encouraging us to acknowledge that all people are different. We all have our own needs, values, personalities, likes and dislikes, we are all unique and this should run through the heart of the decisions and communication strategies that we use. Older people face a raft of complicated societal biases and stereotypes that we all need to acknowledge, but should not allow to influence or determine our attitudes and assumptions about the patient. We need to acknowledge the unique differences of older people and help and guide them to make the best decision for them.

Questions

1. Consider this chapter's content and apply what you have learnt to a recent patient or event. What would you change?
2. How will your approach to older people differ now, considering what you have read?
3. How does this knowledge help to challenge common stereotypes of older age?

References

Brooks L, Manias E, Bloomer M (2018). Culturally sensitive communication in healthcare: a conceptual analysis. *Collegian*, 26(3): 383–391.

Campbell P, et al. (2018). A scoping review of evidence relating to communication failures that lead to patient harm. Available at: https://www.gmc-uk.org/-/media/documents/a-scoping-review-of-evidence-relating-to-communication-failures-that-lead-to-patient-harm_p-80569509.pdf [accessed 6th August 2024].

Centre for Ageing Better (2021). Challenging ageism: A guide to talking about ageing and older age. Available at https://ageing-better.org.uk/publications/challenging-ageism-guide-talking-about-ageing-and-older-age [accessed 6th August 2024].

Eggins S, et al. (2016). *Effective Communication in Clinical Handover: From research to practice*. Berlin: De Greuter.

Eliassen H (2015). Power relations and health care communication in older adulthood: educating recipients and providers. *The Gerontologist*, 56(6): 990–996.

General Medical Council (GMC) (2019). Understanding communication failures involving doctors. Available at: https://www.gmc-uk.org/about/what-we-do-and-why/data-and-research/research-and-insight-archive/understanding-communication-failures-involving-doctors [accessed 6th August 2024].

References

Hewitt-Taylor J (2015). *Developing Person-centred Practice: A practical approach to quality healthcare*. London: Bloomsbury Academic.

Jensen A, et al. (2021). Short communication: opportunities and challenges for early person-centred care for older patients in emergency settings. *International Journal of Environmental Research and Public Health*, 18(23): 12526.

Johnsson A, et al. (2018). Voices used by nurses when communicating with patients and relatives in a department of medicine for older people – an ethnographic study. *Journal of Clinical Nursing*, 27(7–8): e1640–e1650.

Miller A, et al. (2021). Use of seven types of medical jargon by male and female primary care providers at a university health center. *Patient Education and Counselling*, 105(5): 1261–1267.

Milner C, Van Norman K, Milner J (2012). The media's portrayal of ageing. In *Global Population Ageing: Peril or promise?* Working Paper Series. Available at: https://www3.weforum.org/docs/WEF_GAC_GlobalPopulationAgeing_Report_2012.pdf [accessed 6th August 2024].

Naughton C (2018). Patient-centered communication. *Pharmacy*, 6(1): 18.

National Institute for Health and Care Excellence (NICE) (2021). Shared decision making (NICE guideline CG197). Available at: https://www.nice.org.uk/guidance/ng197/chapter/recommendations#communicating-risks-benefits-and-consequences [accessed 6th August 2024].

Pagano M (2015). *Communication Case Studies for Health Care Professionals: An applied approach*. New York: Springer.

Pedersen M, Nielsen V (2019). Bureaucratic decision-making: a multi-method study of gender similarity bias and gender stereotype beliefs. *Public Administration*, 98(2): 424–440.

Silverman J (2016). Information sharing and shared decision making. In *Clinical Communication in Medicine*. Chichester: Wiley Blackwell.

Smith S, Turell S (2019). Perceptions of healthcare experiences: relational and communicative competencies to improve care for LGBT people. *Journal of Social Issue*, 73(3): 637–657.

Stone M, Bazaldua O and Morrow J (2021). Developing health literacy communication practices for medical students. *The Journal of Teaching and Learning Resources*, 17: 11091.

Storlie T (2015). *Person-centred Communication with Older Adults: The professional provider's guide*. San Diego: Elsevier Science and Technology.

Wilson B, et al. (2021). Bridging racial differences in the clinical encounter. How implicit bias and stereotype threat contribute to health care disparities in the dermatology clinic. *International Journal of Women's Dermatology*, 7(2): 139–144.

Chapter 3

Frailty

Carol Robertson and Tom Mallinson

Learning Points

By the end of this chapter, you will:

- Understand the difference between ageing and frailty
- Understand how to screen and identify an individual living with frailty and apply the Clinical Frailty Scale
- Understand the aspects of frailty syndromes
- Understand the components of the comprehensive geriatric assessment.

Case Study

Background: You are an advanced clinical practitioner (ACP) working within an urgent community response (UCR) team. At approximately 09:30 you are contacted by the general practitioner (GP) requesting a visit to a 78-year-old man (Oliver) following an attendance at the local ED last night. Oliver had contacted his doctor this morning as he was struggling to get out of bed. You arrange a visit within two hours.

Presenting Complaint: On arrival, Oliver does not answer the door. Through the window, you see Oliver trying to push a wheeled trolley using only one arm as the other is in a plaster cast. Once in his home, you assist Oliver by linking his arm in support.

History of Presenting Complaint: Oliver informs you that he missed a step yesterday afternoon on his way to the toilet. He tripped on the threshold and fell to the floor. He put his hands out to prevent hitting his head. He was able to get himself off the floor using the step, however his right wrist swelled. He contacted his neighbour and they decided to take him to hospital due to the swelling.

CHAPTER 3 Frailty

An undisplaced distal radius (wrist) fracture was diagnosed and a plaster cast applied. He is struggling to use his walking stick and is experiencing difficulty holding it. He was provided with 'pain killers', but he is worried about taking them with his normal paracetamol.

Past Medical History: Heart failure, chronic kidney disease, cataracts, osteoporosis, hypertension and constipation.

Allergies: No known drug allergies.

Drug History: Alendronic acid (70 mg every Sunday), vitamin D (400 units in morning), Laxido (1–2 sachets as required), paracetamol (1 g four times daily), furosemide (20 mg morning), lisinopril (5 mg morning).

Social History: Oliver lives alone (his husband died two years ago) in a house with a stairlift; the bathroom is upstairs with a toilet downstairs (annex to the kitchen). He has a cleaner weekly for the heavier jobs (for example, hoovering). His daughter does his shopping online, but Oliver tells her what he likes. He usually has microwave meals. He manages his finances, but his daughter also has access to his account in case of an emergency. Oliver stopped driving last year and does not go out alone anymore or even into the garden. His daughter lives in the next town and is caring for her terminally ill husband. Today he is finding everything more difficult due to the injury. He has very helpful neighbours who pop in most days, they take him out in their cars and he enjoys a full social life. He's never smoked and has an occasional glass of wine.

Functional: Oliver uses a walking stick, unless he is wanting to carry items into different rooms: if so, he uses his husband's old, wheeled trolley. He is awaiting a social services needs' assessment as he is finding it increasingly difficult organising his medications and showering.

Assessment

Airway: Maintaining own airway.

Breathing: Speaking in full sentences, with a normal breathing pattern.

Circulation: Well-perfused, no cyanosis. Pulse 70 beats per minute (bpm) and regular, heart sounds normal, no murmurs. Blood pressure 140/88 mmHg initially. Later his lying blood pressure is 138/82 mmHg, standing pressure at 1 minute is 130/84 mmHg, standing at 3 minutes is 142/82. He is not dizzy on standing.

Disabilities: Oliver is FAST-(face, arms, speech, time) negative. He is orientated to place, time and person. He has no dizziness, nausea or vomiting. He tells you his bowels and bladder activity have been normal for him, occasional constipation but no abdominal pain; his abdomen is soft, non-tender and bowel sounds are present. He is 'always needing to pee several times at night' but nothing has changed recently.

Exposure: Apyrexial.

CFS Score: 6.

Cognition: 4AT – 0. Oliver is appropriately dressed for the weather.

Initial Impression: Pain and reduced mobility secondary to wrist injury affecting function, therefore not able to use his usual walking stick. At risk of acute kidney injury and dehydration if he is not able to hydrate as normal due to his reduced function.

Initial Plan: Review medications, prescribe a suitable analgesic, review his bone health, undertake a falls risk assessment, make a therapist referral to assess for appropriate equipment while unable to utilise his wrist, consider a bowel and bladder referral and assess for frailty syndromes.

Introduction

The Office of National Statistics (ONS) (2021) inform us that there are more individuals over 65 years than ever before, accounting for approximately one-sixth of the UK and Wales's population. Approximately 10% of these individuals will be living with frailty, which increases with age (British Geriatrics Society (BGS), 2014). The average life expectancy in the UK between 2018 to 2020 was 79 years for men and 82.9 years for women. However, not everyone over the age of 65 years is living with frailty, likewise, not everyone under 65 is fit and healthy.

Within health and social care, we can become biased in our views of older people because they are often in crisis when we meet them. Individuals living with frailty are among the highest users of health and social care services and make up the highest proportion of unintentional attendances at hospitals (Mytton, 2012). Understanding frailty and the impact on an individual is essential. Furthermore, primary and community care providers (prevention, crisis response, intermediate care) are fundamental to accomplishing national goals to assist more people living with frailty to live well at or nearer to home (NHS Providers, 2024). Ambulance clinicians are the bridge to getting the individuals to the appropriate teams – the right place, at the right time.

Oliver is living with moderate frailty. He requires help with all outdoor activities and with keeping house; however, he can normally complete his personal ADLs, such as washing and dressing, without help.

Oliver demonstrates how a person living with frailty is affected by a minor event. A fractured wrist is more of an inconvenience for younger people, but because Oliver requires his right hand to hold his stick, it immediately impedes his normal function. Oliver would benefit from a holistic approach assessing his risks associated with living with moderate frailty including his reduced function, balance, mobility and environmental issues (including socioeconomic factors) which will ensure he is safe within his home. Furthermore, he requires an evaluation of his pain including a medication review to ensure all medicines are essential. Exploration of any medical and psychological concerns should be considered.

Socioeconomic Factors

There are approximately two million retirees living in relative poverty (Dixon, 2020). Lower area incomes and higher area material deprivation is associated with higher levels of frailty (Mangin et al., 2023). Frailty often accompanies comorbidities; however, a considerable correlation was identified in those with more than three long-term diseases, smoking, obesity and socioeconomic deprivation (Hanlon et al., 2018). It is important to have an awareness of the individual's socioeconomic status to allow a thorough examination of their medical needs as well as consideration of how this may affect their care needs.

What is Frailty?

While clinical frailty is not caused by a single pathology, it is a key concern in modern health and is often recognised in patients presenting to healthcare professionals with one or multiple issues. These common presentations, known as 'frailty syndromes', include delirium, immobility, falls, incontinence and susceptibility to the side effects of medications. Many of these elements of frailty cannot be covered in one chapter with many subjects commanding their own chapters (Chapter 8: Falls, Chapter 6: Polypharmacy and Medicines Review) or extensive discussion within chapters (for example, immobility, vision, orthostatic hypotension (OH)). Furthermore, social isolation and loneliness are not among the five frailty syndromes; however, living with recurrent falls, immobility or incontinence can lead to social isolation, which often precedes loneliness. Loneliness can compound the probability of physical frailty (Gale et al., 2018).

Defining frailty as a clinical entity is challenging and definitions vary. Xue has defined it as a clinical syndrome of

> 'increased vulnerability, resulting from ageing-associated decline in reserve and function, across multiple physiologic systems, such that the ability to cope with every day or acute stressors is compromised.'
>
> (Xue, 2011)

The common theme is that individuals living with frailty can demonstrate increased susceptibility to side effects of medications, falls, delirium, immobility or incontinence following an acute event (Turner, 2014) often resulting in decline (BGS, 2018; Clegg et al., 2013; Oo et al., 2013).

Frailty Measurement and Screening Tools

It is important to be able to recognise those individuals who are defined as living with frailty because, being more susceptible to 'frailty syndromes', they are at increased risk of an admission to hospital or long-term care (NHS England, 2024). Notably, frailty is a complicated geriatric sequence which must be considered when any older adult has an acute event (Oo et al., 2013).

Frailty Measurement and Screening Tools

Frailty tools use either the phenotype measure or a deficit model. Fried et al.'s phenotype model linked making a frailty diagnosis to the presence of at least three of these measurable parameters: low grip strength, low energy, slowed walking speed, low physical activity and/or unintentional weight loss (2001). A more recent approach to defining frailty is the deficit model established by Rockwood et al. (2005). The Clinical Frailty Scale (CFS) was one of many frailty tools applied to over 2,300 older patients; the outcome of this research confirmed the CFS was able to forecast the risk of institutional care or death (Rockwood et al., 2005). The more issues, the higher the risks of frailty.

Clinical frailty correlates well to various patient outcomes such as length of in-patient stay, readmission rates and in-patient mortality (Table 3.1). Therefore, early identification of clinical frailty at both an individual and population level can be hugely beneficial for decision making in relation to clinical management of a patient and when designing or funding whole systems. Within the UK, the increased length of in-patient stay has projected healthcare costs (associated with frailty) of £5.9 billion annually (Heaven et al., 2019).

Table 3.1 Clinical Frailty Scale and its correlation to secondary care outcomes.

Clinical Frailty Scale Grading	Length of Hospital Stay (Days)	In-Patient Mortality
1	4	2%
2	5	2%
3	7	2%
4	8	3%
5	10	4%
6	12	6%
7	13	11%
8	12	24%
9	10	31%

Source: Adapted from Specialised Clinical Frailty Network, 2023.

CHAPTER 3 Frailty

Assessing and quantifying frailty is a significant challenge. Several tools for assessing clinical frailty are in existence, such as the Electronic Frailty Index (eFI) developed by Clegg et al. (2016) in England. The eFI compiles the individual's health deficits from their electronic record; there are 36 deficits and 2,000 codes which incorporate clinical signs, symptoms, diseases, disabilities and abnormal test values. It has been validated in over 900,000 patients (Clegg et al., 2016). It stratifies risk as mild, moderate or severely frail (Clegg et al., 2016). Within Scotland, the Scottish Patients at Risk of Readmission and Admission (SPARRA) is utilised. Both of these tools are applied at a population level, where large datasets can be assessed to inform health policy and to plan preventive or anticipatory care regionally or nationally. However, many of these tools require a clinician to administer specific physical tests such as the Timed Up and Go Test (TUGT) or the frailty phenotype, which requires information such as grip strength or gait speed and calculations of weekly energy expenditure by the patient.

ED front-door frailty screening is essential (Buurman et al., 2021; NHS Rightcare, 2019; NHSE, 2024), because recognising frailty can help us to understand the consequences an insult has on a person (Moody, 2017; Turner, 2014). The CFS is advocated for use within EDs alongside the National Early Warning Score 2 (NEWS2) and the 4 'A's Test (4AT) within 30 minutes of arrival; additionally for patients with a CFS score of more than 6, a comprehensive geriatric assessment (CGA) should be initiated (NHSE, 2024).

There are also several screening tools, which have a focus on identifying frailty, rather than stratifying or quantifying the degree of frailty. Such screening tools include Think Frailty, the FiND Questionnaire, Gérontopôle or the FRESH-Screening tool. In clinical practice, a tool which enables a degree of stratification of frailty can be far more useful when there is a need to inform decisions around care planning or clinical management (Table 3.2).

Applying a Frailty Tool

The CFS developed by Professor Ken Rockwood (Figure 3.1) is perhaps the most user-friendly assessment tool and is commonly used across the NHS (Green et al., 2018). It was developed to enable a way to capture the whole level of frailty or fitness of an older person following an assessment by an experienced clinician (Rockwood et al., 2005). It enables a rapid assessment of a patient's condition, but it does rely on a degree of clinical judgement and although good inter-rater reliability has been demonstrated (Young and Smithard, 2020), concern remains around its use by novice clinicians. To this end additional tools such as the Clinical Frailty Scale Classification Tree (Theou et al., 2021) and the CFS app (Acute Frailty Network, 2023) have been developed.

However, despite being well validated and demonstrated to be reliable, there are still some common pitfalls that need to be avoided when assessing frailty using the CFS. The tool was designed to assess someone's baseline status, specifically their usual level of function and health approximately **two weeks before** the onset of an acute illness. Therefore, it is important to understand their normal level of function and medical background, rather than basing the assessment on how they may present when acutely unwell.

Frailty Measurement and Screening Tools

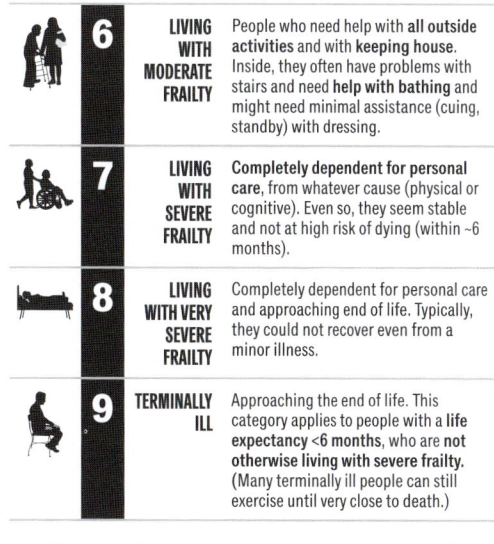

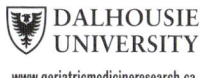

Figure 3.1 The Clinical Frailty Scale.
Source: Reprinted from 'Using the Clinical Frailty Scale in Allocating Scarce Health Care Resources' by Rockwood K and Theou O, 2020. Canadian Geriatrics Journal. 23(3), 211. Copyright 2020 by Kenneth Rockwood. Reprinted with permission.

A caveat to this is a patient presenting in what appears to be a dying phase, where they may score 9, 'terminally ill', despite a much better recent baseline. Be careful not to escalate a person's frailty score simply due to multimorbidity. A patient may have diabetes, epilepsy and asthma and still score 1 and be 'very fit'. Concurrent dementia can make frailty scoring harder. A rough rule of thumb is that mild, moderate and severe dementia map across to scores of 5, 6 and 7, respectively. Finally, the Rockwood Scale is only validated for individuals aged 65 and over and should not be used for younger patients or those with long-term disabilities (Rockwood et al., 2005).

A current issue with frailty screening in prehospital care is that no screening tools have been validated to date. However, a recent scoping review identified that six different frailty screening tools are in use throughout the UK by prehospital clinicians, with paramedics acknowledging frailty assessments to be achievable and essential (Alshibani et al., 2023). Likewise, many UCR and community teams are using frailty screening.

CHAPTER 3 Frailty

Labelling frailty without identifying a level runs the risk of 'frailism' standing in as a subtle form of ageism (Rockwood, 2021). Furthermore, distinguishing older individuals who are living with frailty from those who are not frail should be a crucial aspect of any healthcare assessment, especially if the potential outcome is an invasive procedure or potentially harmful medication (Clegg et al., 2013). Below, Majorie and Morag will demonstrate the importance of identifying an individual's baseline. Compare the two women in Table 3.2 and answer the questions below.

Table 3.2 Frailty case study.

Patient 1	Patient 2
Marjorie is a 68-year-old woman and an active member of the local heritage society, often leading walks around the village and surrounding countryside to discuss sites of historical significance. She takes an aspirin a day (of her own volition) and started ramipril last year for mild hypertension.	Morag is a 68-year-old woman. Five years ago, she had a stroke which left her with significant unilateral weakness and requiring carers three times a day. It is believed the stroke occurred in relation to unchecked hypertension, hypercholesterolaemia and perhaps underlying vascular dementia.
Today she has phoned an ambulance after tripping over her cat in the garden. Clinically, she has a fracture to her neck of femur.	While her carers were transferring her from her bed to a chair today, she slipped and appears to have fractured her hip.
What is her CFS score likely to be?	What is her CFS score likely to be?
What do you think the 30-day and 1-year mortality (%) will be for a patient with this CFS score?	What do you think the 30-day and 1-year mortality (%) will be for a patient with this CFS score?
Marjorie probably has a CFS score of 2 (fit).	Morag probably has a CFS score of 6 or 7 (living with moderate or severe frailty).
Marjorie probably has a 1.5% mortality in the next 30 days and a 4% in the next year.	Morag has an approximate 7–14% mortality within 30 days and a 1-year mortality of 40%.

Source: Mortality data from Narula et al., 2020.

Now apply the CFS to Oliver's (our patient from the case study's) function from **two weeks** previously. Use either Figure 3.1 or download the CFS app. Did you also conclude that Oliver is 'living with moderate frailty' (CFS score 6), which indicates to 'actively seek out and manage geriatric syndromes'?

A study of patients over the age of 80 diagnosed with fractures revealed that advancing frailty was more prevalent in women; however, men had a higher mortality rate (Ravindrarajah et al., 2018). Figure 3.2 demonstrates the impact a minor injury or illness can have on an older person and the balance between independent and dependent.

Frailty Syndromes

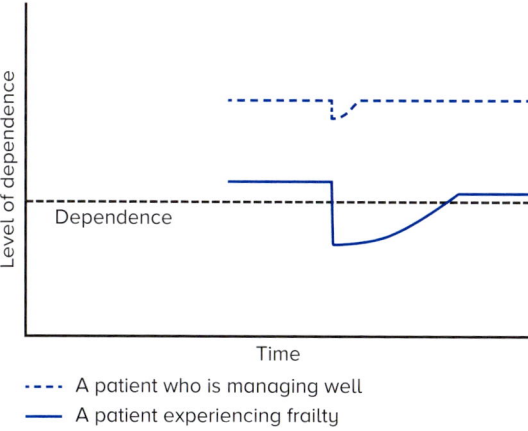

Figure 3.2 The impact a minor illness or injury can have on a person living with frailty compared to those who are well.
Source: Based on Clegg et al., 2013.

Frailty Syndromes

There are five recognised frailty syndromes: falls, immobility, delirium, incontinence and the susceptibility to the side effects of medications (Turner, 2014). If your patient presents with one of these, it suggests that the patient may be living with frailty. However, as previously mentioned, not everyone over 65 years is frail.

Older people living with frailty requiring urgent medical attention should not be underestimated. Timely identification and management of frailty syndromes and their underlying source in the acute situation delivers better patient outcomes (within 24 hours); delayed care can lead to increased mortality, irreversible damage, extended periods of hospitalisation and potentially delayed discharge (Frailty Fulcrum, 2016). Many patients may present with more than one non-specific problem: for example, a fall when rushing to the toilet due to their incontinence, pain causing immobility; analgesic's side effects potentially causing acute confusion (delirium). Furthermore, a reduction in mobility might result from a cardiac event, rather than a worsening of arthritis, even in the absence of classic symptoms. Therefore, a thorough and cautious clinical evaluation is essential (Frailty Fulcrum, 2016).

Delirium

Delirium is not a disease, but rather a symptom defined as 'the onset of sudden confusion' (NHS, 2021). Delirium can be constant or fluctuate over hours, days, weeks or months and can present in several ways: hypoactive, hyperactive and mixed (NICE, 2021; Preston and Wilkinson, 2016a). It can manifest as hallucinations, disorientation, difficulty concentrating or comprehending questions and personality changes (irritable or withdrawn). It can be distressing for both patients and their loved ones (BGS, 2021). It can be difficult differentiating between dementias and deliriums, but it is usually the acute onset of symptoms which distinguishes delirium. It is worth noting that delirium can happen to anyone of any age when experiencing illness and/or prolonged hospital stays.

Hyperactive delirium (characterised by increased psychomotor activity) can involve altered insight, including hallucinations, restlessness, distrust and/or aggression (NICE, 2023). The patient may feel afraid or threatened triggering flight (Rahman, 2020). In contrast individuals with hypoactive delirium may present with reduced alertness, depression, weepiness or drowsiness (NICE, 2023). It may be difficult to engage the patient in conversation as they may demonstrate inattention or slower than normal cognition or processing. Furthermore, it may be challenging to encourage food and fluids, potentially leading to dehydration and malnutrition which can exacerbate delirium. Rahman (2020) notes that this situation can often resemble the presentation of end-of-life patients. Lastly, mixed delirium may present as a combination of the above. It is often missed due to the variety of signs and symptoms (NICE, 2023) therefore, even when you think you have identified the causative factor, keep exploring as it is often multifaceted (Robertson, 2022). Causes of delirium can be recalled through the mnemonic PINCHES ME (CGA Toolkit, n.d.):

- **P**ain
- **I**nfection
- **N**utrition
- **C**onstipation
- **H**ydration
- **E**ndocrine and **E**lectrolyte
- **S**troke
- **M**edication and Alcohol
- **E**nvironmental.

Assessment and diagnosis can be assisted with screening tools for delirium of which there are several. NICE (2021) suggests completing a cognitive assessment from one of the following: 4AT, the short Confusion Assessment Method (CAM) or the Diagnostic and Statistical Manual of Mental Disorders (DSM-5) criteria. The 4AT is highly specific and sensitive and has been validated in studies involving more than 5,000 patients (MacLullich, 2023). The 4AT comprises four sections (alertness, cognition, attention and fluctuating or increased confusion) with questions and observations, including explanatory notes.

Confusion screen blood tests are often required. These usually include a full blood count (FBC), urea and electrolytes (U&E), bone, liver, B12, folate, vitamin D, magnesium, thyroid and glucose tests to determine deficiencies and imbalances. Additionally, the patient may need specific investigations to rule out certain pathologies, for example a chest X-ray for possible pneumonia or a midstream urine analysis to detect urinary infections. It is worth noting that a positive 'dip' is not confirmation of an infection in older people. Approximately 50% of older people (and the majority of those with catheters) will have bacteria within the bladder and/or urine without an infection; this is 'asymptomatic bacteriuria' which may cause a positive urine dipstick, but is not detrimental (Public Health England, 2020).

Management of delirium should be focussed on treating the cause and managing triggers. For example, if caused by an acute infection, consider antibiotics; if caused by constipation, treat with laxatives; if there are environmental causes, try to familiarise and reorientate the individual (always ensure correct lighting, glasses and hearing aids are worn, reduce unnecessary changes, for example moving rooms in a care home or wards in a hospital). NICE (2021) suggests that out of hospital care may be appropriate; however, it is important to understand the cause and be able to treat it within the community, while ensuring the patient is safe with appropriate supervision and follow-up (NICE, 2021). It is essential those caring for the individual can quickly identify and escalate the situation if the patient deteriorates. Furthermore, a person with delirium will also be more susceptible to the other frailty syndromes, so pharmacological treatments should be avoided if possible (NICE, 2021).

Susceptibility to the Side Effects of Medications

This is a significant issue for older people living with frailty and can also be a cause of delirium and/or withdrawal (Rahman, 2020). A detailed review of medications is required with a focus on deprescribing harmful or unnecessary drugs (Nickel et al., 2021). Chapter 6: Polypharmacy and Medicines Review discusses medications, deprescribing and polypharmacy in detail.

Falls

Falls are very common and approximately half of those over 80 and a third of those over 65 will fall each year within the UK (Office for Health Improvement and Disparities (OHID), 2022). Falls from standing height are the most common cause of major trauma in older adults (Trauma Audit and Research Network, 2017). Chapter 8: Falls discusses risk factors, the importance of differentiating between pre-syncopal, syncopal and non-syncopal events and the need to identify both intrinsic and extrinsic causes and contributing factors. Older people presenting with significant injuries are covered in Chapter 9: Major Trauma.

Immobility

Immobility can present acutely and is often secondary to illness or injury. Exploring an individual's baseline mobility/self-care capability, plus their acuity of deterioration is essential (Nickel et al., 2021). Understanding a patient's baseline frailty level can be extremely beneficial to understanding the acute change. Immobility is discussed in more detail in Chapter 7: Activities of Daily Living.

Incontinence

Continence requires not only a working urinary system, including the bladder and sphincter, but also cognition, ability, movement and a suitable environment (Woodford, 2022). Incontinence is the unintended passing of urine or faeces. It is essential to understand if this is a new or ongoing symptom (Preston and Wilkinson, 2016b).

Urinary incontinence affects millions of people and there are several different types (Preston and Wilkinson, 2016b; NHS, 2023):

- Stress incontinence: leakage when coughing or laughing.
- Urge incontinence (also referred to as overactive bladder): urinary leakage and an intense urge to urinate (it is possible to have stress and urge incontinence together).
- Overflow incontinence (chronic urinary retention): inability to fully empty the bladder causing frequent leakage (usually in men).
- Total incontinence: inability of the bladder to store urine leading to frequent leaking or constantly passing urine.
- Functional: outside of the urinary system, such as mobility, dexterity or cognition.

Cortical input to control contraction and relaxation of external sphincters, plus bladder motor control, is essential for continence, but ageing can also contribute, due to the functional volume of the bladder reducing, yet the residual capacity expanding (Woodford, 2022). Additionally, healthy older people can produce more urine overnight. Peripheral oedema, certain medications or heart failure can also increase night-time urine production, leading to reabsorption when supine (Woodford, 2022). There are numerous stages to physically getting to a toilet or commode, such as: cognition (knowing you need to go), function (ability to walk, sit upright and stand) and dexterity (removing clothing and using toilet paper) (Preston and Wilkinson, 2016b). One study identified that older people with symptoms of an overactive bladder have higher levels of decreased function, multimorbidity and polypharmacy (Ganz et al., 2016).

Examination is crucial for identifying acute and treatable underlying pathologies, such as symptomatic genitourinary prolapse, enlarged prostate, genitourinary syndrome of menopause and faecal loading. Additionally, assessing pelvic floor function is important (BGS, 2019a). Many people find the subject of incontinence stigmatising and may choose not to disclose willingly. Therefore, asking patients about their continence is important. Assisting with toileting can be difficult, but it is important to support patients to remain continent (Woodford, 2022). Often mobility, position and hydration will help with bowel and bladder issues however intermittent catheters are used for acute retention, management in the very unwell or following a specific procedure. An indwelling catheter (long term) may be considered, but may require specialist input. Always consider a referral to a bladder and bowel service as their knowledge of treatments and products can make significant changes for individuals.

The Comprehensive Geriatric Assessment (CGA)

A CGA explores not only medical, but also previous and current function including cognition, continence, ADLs, social network and their ideas, concerns and expectations (Conroy et al., 2019; Skills for Health, 2018). The CGA is advocated in acute illness to examine probable frailty syndromes; however, the suitability of interventions and investigations which do not add value needs to be carefully considered. This allows an understanding of what the patient's priorities are while considering their prognosis (Buurman et al., 2021; Conroy et al., 2018; 2019). Below, Figure 3.3 demonstrates the components of a CGA.

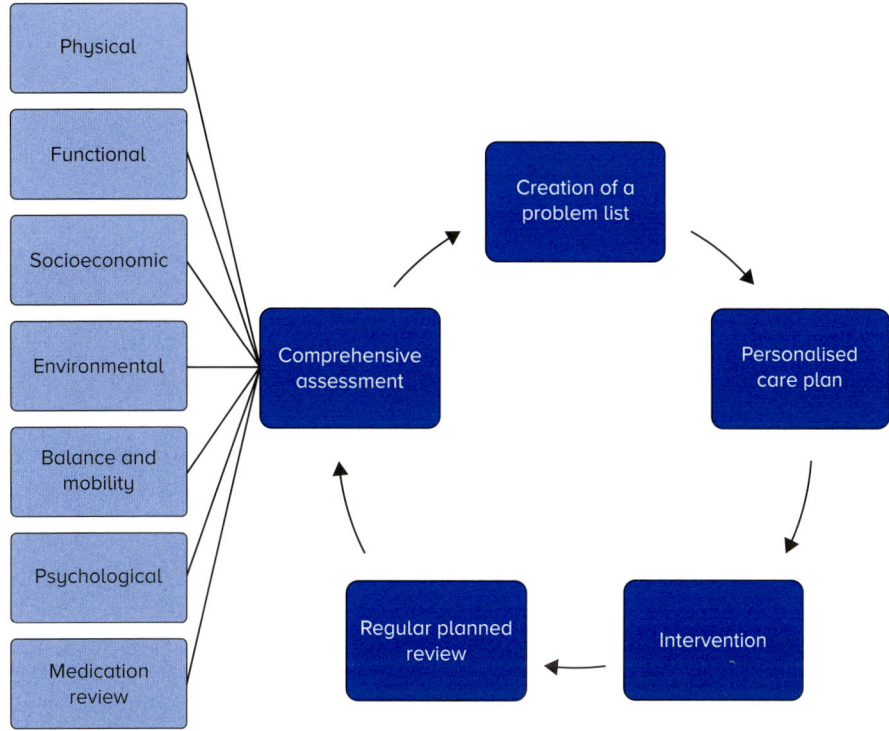

Figure 3.3 The elements of a CGA.
Source: Adapted from the British Geriatrics Society, 2019b.

A toolkit has been produced by the BGS to aid the use of CGAs in primary care with detailed information regarding the four overarching elements: physical assessment, functional, social and environmental assessment, psychological components and medication reviews (BGS, 2019a). The CGA approach to older people's care is an underlying process to enable a team working towards a shared common goal (Hogervorst et al., 2021; Skills for Health, 2018). The level of care and input will be determined by the patient's level of frailty. For example, a CGA is not usually required for individuals living with mild frailty (NHSE, 2023), but it is recommended for those living with moderate frailty to address all aspects of their health and well-being (NHSE, 2023). As well as a CGA, the focus for those living with severe frailty should be on evaluating their care needs and developing a care plan that prioritises the individual's goals (NHSE, 2023). Importantly the CGA is not just for geriatricians, but can be conducted by an MDT with the relevant expertise to focus on frailty (Buurman et al., 2021). The core assessment team can include a variety of healthcare professionals with the circumstances and location determining the depth of your assessment and/or initial care plan.

CHAPTER 3 Frailty

The CGA is the gold standard approach for improving care for older people in acute hospitals (Conroy et al., 2019) and NHSE are advocating for a CGA to be initiated within 30 minutes of arrival at ED for all patients with a frailty score of more than 6 (NHS Improvement, NHSE, the Ambulatory Emergency Care Network and the Acute Frailty Network, 2019). Therefore, any prehospital information gained may help contribute towards a CGA completed by an MDT or geriatrician. For example, the social, functional and environmental factors observed and documented during home visits or ambulance call-outs may be the only insight into how the patient is managing at home. These factors may also contribute towards discharge planning or advance care planning for patients in hospital or intermediate care.

In essence a CGA is a holistic approach that necessitates actions from the assessors, leading to specific outcomes for the individual (Buurman et al., 2021).

Advance Care Planning

The aim of advance care planning is to facilitate an individual to receive clinical care that meets their choices during serious and chronic health conditions (Sudore et al., 2017). The *Silver Book II* advocates that advance care planning should be a systematic practice (following or prompted by an acute episode) to explore an individual's care goals (Nickel et al., 2021).

Individuals with early cognitive deterioration can plan for a variety of potential choices during their illness path (Linger et al., 2008). Many older people living with Alzheimer's disease have experienced poorer outcomes towards the end of their lives compared to those with a single condition. This has been partially attributed to health professionals not identifying the last year of a patient's life (Care Quality Commission, 2016). Chapter 10: Palliative and End-of life Care discusses advance care plans in further detail.

Conclusion

This chapter has demonstrated the importance of screening for frailty to enable recognition of people who are at risk of adverse events such as not returning to their baseline following a minor illness or injury. Screening for frailty prehospitally can assist in handovers to ED, falls teams, GPs, therapists and further care as it is a common and communal language. Applying the frailty score does not require training, with the easiest resource being the CFS app. It is imperative when using the CFS tool that you base the frailty score on the patient's usual level of function and health at least two weeks prior to the onset of illness.

The significance of recognising frailty syndromes, such as in Oliver's case, and the need for a holistic approach with a CGA involving targeted actions and outcomes (Buurman et al., 2021), can be substantial. Additionally, it is crucial to document an individual's baseline function, social situation, continence, cognition and environment. This documentation aids in discharge planning, CGAs and advance care planning and helps understanding of deterioration and prioritising the individual's wishes.

Resources for Your Patients and Their Family or Carers

> **Questions**
>
> 1. Consider this chapter's content and apply what you have learnt to a recent patient or family member. What frailty syndromes were present?
> 2. Can you think of any recent patients who may have demonstrated a hypoactive delirium?
> 3. Think holistically, what systems or support are available when you next encounter a similar patient? Who do you want in your MDT?

Further Resources

- British Geriatrics Society (2021). *Silver Book II. Quality care for older people with urgent care need.* Available at: https://www.bgs.org.uk/resources/resource-series/silver-book-ii
- British Geriatrics Society (2023). *Frailty elearning free to all.* Available at: https://www.bgs.org.uk/policy-and-media/frailty-elearning-free-to-all
- Geeky Medics (2024). *Medical education platform.* Available at: https://geekymedics.com/
- Health Education England, NHS England and Skills for Health (2018). *Frailty: A framework of core capabilities.* Available at: https://www.skillsforhealth.org.uk/wp-content/uploads/2021/01/Frailty-framework.pdf
- The Hearing Aid Podcasts. *Podcast series.* Available at: http://thehearingaidpodcasts.org.uk/
- NHS Rightcare (2019). *Frailty Toolkit. Optimising a frailty system.* Available at: https://www.england.nhs.uk/rightcare/wp-content/uploads/sites/40/2019/07/frailty-toolkit-june-2019-v1.pdf
- World guidelines for falls prevention and management for older adults: a global initiative: https://academic.oup.com/ageing/article/51/9/afac205/6730755?login=false

Resources for Your Patients and Their Family or Carers

- Age UK: https://www.ageuk.org.uk/
- British Red Cross: for help and support such as loaning equipment and transport for essential healthcare journeys, help with everyday tasks, companionship and rebuilding confidence; https://www.redcross.org.uk/get-help/get-support-at-home.
- Parkinson's UK: Helpline 0808 800 0303; https://www.parkinsons.org.uk/.
- Royal Volunteering Society (RVS): Aid with collecting shopping, medication or other essential supplies; 0808 196 3646 0800-2000; https://www.royalvoluntaryservice.org.uk/our-services/social-activities

- Silverline: A helpline for older people; 0800 4 70 80 90; https://www.thesilverline.org.uk/what-we-do/
- Social prescribers/care connectors: available via GP or local authority websites.

References

Acute Frailty Network (2023). Clinical Frailty Scale (CFS) app. Available at: https://play.google.com/store/apps/details?id=com.clinicalfrailtyscale&pli=1 [accessed 28th September 2023].

Alshibani A, et al. (2023). Frailty identification in prehospital care: a scoping review of the literature. *Open Access Emergency Medicine*, 15: 227–239.

British Geriatrics Society (BGS) (2014). Fit for frailty – consensus best practice guidance for the care of older people living in community and outpatient settings – a report from the British Geriatrics Society 2014. Available at: https://www.bgs.org.uk/sites/default/files/content/resources/files/2018-05-23/fff_full.pdf [accessed 27th May 2024.].

British Geriatrics Society (BGS) (2018). Frailty: what's it all about? Available at: https://www.bgs.org.uk/resources/frailty-what%E2%80%99s-it-all-about [accessed 28th September 2023].

British Geriatrics Society (BGS) (2019a). CGA in primary care settings: patients presenting with urinary incontinence. Available at: https://www.bgs.org.uk/resources/16-cga-in-primary-care-settings-patients-presenting-with-urinary-incontinence [accessed 28th September 2023].

British Geriatrics Society (BGS) (2019b). Comprehensive Geriatric Assessment Toolkit for Primary Care Practitioners. Available at: https://www.bgs.org.uk/sites/default/files/content/resources/files/2019-03-12/CGA%20Toolkit%20for%20Primary%20Care%20Practitioners_0.pdf [accessed 7th August 2024]

British Geriatrics Society (BGS) (2021). BGS launches new comprehensive delirium resource. Available at: https://www.bgs.org.uk/policy-and-media/bgs-launches-new-comprehensive-delirium-resource [accessed 27th May 2024].

Buurman B, Martin F, Conroy S (2021). *Silver Book II: Holistic assessment of older people*. Available at: https://www.bgs.org.uk/resources/silver-book-ii-holistic-assessment-of-older-people [accessed 28th September 2023].

Care Quality Commission (2016). A different ending: addressing inequalities in end of life care. Overview report. Available at: https://www.cqc.org.uk/sites/default/files/20160505%20CQC_EOLC_OVERVIEW_FINAL_3.pdf [accessed 28th September 2023].

CGA Toolkit Plus (n.d.). Delirium. Available at: https://www.cgakit.com/p-2-delirium [accessed 28th September 2023].

Clegg A, et al. (2013). Frailty in elderly people. *The Lancet*, 381(9868): 752–762.

Clegg A, et al. (2016). Development and validation of an electronic frailty index using routine primary care electronic health record data. *Age and Ageing*, 45(3): 353–360.

Conroy SP (2018). Hospital wide comprehensive geriatric assessment (HoW-CGA): Overview. Available at: https://www.bgs.org.uk/resources/hospital-wide-comprehensive-geriatric-assessment-how-cga-overview [accessed 28th September 2023].

Conroy SP, et al. (2019). Comprehensive geriatric assessment for frail older people in acute hospitals: the HoW-CGA mixed-methods study. Available at: https://www.ncbi.nlm.nih.gov/books/NBK540056/pdf/Bookshelf_NBK540056.pdf [accessed 28th September 2023].

Dixon A (2020). *The Age of Ageing Better*. London: Bloomsbury.

Frailty Fulcrum (2016). The frailty syndromes: managing frailty in acute settings. Available at: https://www.frailtytoolkit.org/the-frailty-syndromes/ [accessed 28th September 2023].

Fried LP, et al. (2001). Cardiovascular health study collaborative research group. *The Journals of Gerontology: Series A, Biological Sciences and Medical Sciences*, 56(3): M146–156.

Gale CR, Westbury L, Cooper C (2018). Social isolation and loneliness as risk factors for the progression of frailty: the English longitudinal study of ageing. *Age and Ageing*, 47(3): 392–397.

References

Ganz ML, et al. (2016). Real-world characteristics of elderly patients with overactive bladder in the United States. *Current Medical Research and Opinion*, 32(12): 1997–2005.

Green J, Kirby K, Hope S (2018). Ambulance clinicians' perceptions, assessment and management of frailty: thematic analysis of focus groups. *British Paramedic Journal*, 3(3): 23–33.

Hanlon P, et al. (2018). Frailty and pre-frailty in middle-aged and older adults and its association with multimorbidity and mortality: a prospective analysis of 493 737 UK Biobank participants. *Lancet Public Health*, 3(7): e323–332.

Heaven A, et al. (2019). Community ageing research 75+ study (CARE75+): an experimental ageing and frailty research cohort. *British Medical Journal Open*, 9(3): e026744.

Hogervorst VM, et al. (2021). Emergency department management of older people living with frailty: a guide for emergency practitioners. *British Medical Journal*, 38(9): 724–729.

Linger HH, et al. (2008). Frequency and correlates of advance planning among cognitively impaired older adults. *The American Journal of Geriatric Psychiatry*, 16(8): 643–649.

MacLullich A (2023). 4AT. Rapid clinical test for delirium. Available at: https://www.the4at.com/ [accessed 28th September 2023].

Mangin D, et al. (2023). Association between frailty, chronic conditions and socioeconomic status in community-dwelling older adults attending primary care: a cross-sectional study using practice-based research network data. *British Medical Journal Open*, 13: e066269.

Moody D (2017). 'Finding frailty': system benefits of frailty identification. NHS England. The 3rd National Frailty Conference, Leeds. Available at: https://static1.squarespace.com/static/5b5f1d4e9d5abb9699cb8a75/t/5b911645562fa7cd9913a6b4/1536235082006/moody_finding_frailty.pdf [accessed 28th September 2023].

Mytton OT, et al. (2012). Avoidable acute hospital admission in older people. *British Journal of Healthcare Management*, 18(11): 597–603.

Narula S, et al. (2020). Clinical Frailty Scale is a good predictor of mortality after proximal femur fracture: A cohort study of 30-day and one-year mortality. *Bone Joint Open*, 1(8): 443–449.

National Institute for Health and Care Excellence (NICE) (2021). Delirium: how should I assess a person with suspected delirium? Available at: https://cks.nice.org.uk/topics/delirium/diagnosis/assessment/ [accessed 28th September 2023].

National Institute for Health and Care Excellence (NICE) (2023). Delirium: Prevention, diagnosis and management in hospital and long-term care (NICE guideline NG176). Available at: https://www.nice.org.uk/guidance/ng176 [accessed 27th May 2024].

NHS (2021). Sudden confusion (delirium). Available at: https://www.nhs.uk/conditions/confusion/ [accessed 28th September 2023].

NHS (2023). Urinary incontinence. Available at: https://www.nhs.uk/conditions/urinary-incontinence/ [accessed 29th September 2023].

NHS England (2023). Living with frailty. Available at: https://www.england.nhs.uk/ourwork/clinical-policy/older-people/frailty/living-with-frailty/ [accessed 28th September 2023].

NHS England (2024). FRAIL strategy. Available at: https://www.england.nhs.uk/long-read/frail-strategy/ [accessed 12th April 2024].

NHS Improvement, NHS England, the Ambulatory Emergency Care Network and the Acute Frailty Network (2019). Same-day acute frailty services. Available at: https://www.england.nhs.uk/wp-content/uploads/2021/02/SDEC_guide_frailty_May_2019_update.pdf [accessed 29th September 2023].

NHS Providers (2024). Community network. Supporting people living with frailty. The case for supporting people with frailty in the community. Available at: https://nhsproviders.org/community-network-supporting-people-living-with-frailty/the-case-for-supporting-people-with-frailty-in-the-community [accessed 12th April 2024].

NHS RightCare (2019). NHS RightCare: Frailty toolkit: optimising a frailty system. Available at: https://www.england.nhs.uk/rightcare/wp-content/uploads/sites/40/2019/07/frailty-toolkit-june-2019-v1.pdf [accessed 29th September 2023].

CHAPTER 3 Frailty

Nickel C, et al. (2021). *Silver Book II: Geriatric syndromes*. Available at: https://www.bgs.org.uk/resources/silver-book-ii-geriatric-syndromes [accessed 28th September 2023].

Office for Health Improvement and Disparities (OHID) (2022). *Falls: Applying All Our Health*. Available at https://www.gov.uk/government/publications/falls-applying-all-our-health/falls-applying-all-our-health [accessed 29th September 2023].

Office for National Statistics (ONS) (2021). Population and household estimates, England and Wales: Census 2021. Available at: https://www.ons.gov.uk/peoplepopulationandcommunity/populationandmigration/populationestimates/bulletins/populationandhouseholdestimatesenglandandwales/census2021 [accessed 12th April 2024].

Oo MT, et al. (2013). Assessing frailty in the acute medical admission of elderly patients. *Royal College of Physicians Edinburgh*, 43: 301–308.

Preston J, Wilkinson I (2016a). The MDTea podcast. Episode 1.2 Delirium. Available at: http://thehearingaidpodcasts.org.uk/episode-1-2-delirium/ [accessed 27th September 2023].

Preston J, Wilkinson I (2016b). The MDTea Podcast. Episode 1.3 Urinary incontinence. Available at: http://thehearingaidpodcasts.org.uk/episode-1-3-urinary-incontinence/ [accessed 27th September 2023].

Public Health England (2020). Diagnosis of urinary tract infections: quick reference tool for primary care for consultation and local adaptation. Available at: https://www.gov.uk/government/consultations/urinary-tract-infection-diagnostic-tools-for-primary-care/diagnosis-of-urinary-tract-infections-quick-reference-tools-for-primary-care [accessed 12th April 2024].

Rahman S (2020). *Essentials of Delirium. Everything you really need to know for working in delirium care*. London: Routledge.

Ravindrarajah R, et al. (2018). Incidence and mortality of fractures by frailty level over 80 years of age: cohort study using UK electronic health records. *British Medical Journal Open*, 8: e018836.

Robertson C (2022). Delirium and dementia. In *Mental Health Care in Paramedic Practice*, Rolfe U and Partlow D (eds.) Bridgwater, Class Professional Publishing: 137–148.

Rockwood K, et al. (2005). A global clinical measure of fitness and frailty in elderly people. *Canadian Medical Association Journal*, 173(5): 489–495.

Rockwood K (2021). Silver Book II: Frailty. Available at: https://www.bgs.org.uk/resources/silver-book-ii-frailty [accessed 28th September 2023].

Rockwood K, Theou O (2020). Clinical Frailty Scale. Available at: https://www.dal.ca/sites/gmr/our-tools/clinical-frailty-scale.html [accessed 29th Sept 2023].

Skills for Health (2018). Frailty: a framework of core capabilities. Available at: https://www.skillsforhealth.org.uk/wp-content/uploads/2021/01/Frailty-framework.pdf [accessed 3rd February 2024].

Specialised Clinical Frailty Network (2023). Clinical Frailty Scale. Available at: https://www.scfn.org.uk/clinical-frailty-scale [accessed 5 September 2024].

Sudore RL, et al. (2017). Defining advance care planning for adults: a consensus definition from a multidisciplinary Delphi panel. *Journal of Pain and Symptom Management*, 53(5): 821–832.

Theou O, et al. (2021). A classification tree to assist with routine scoring of the Clinical Frailty Scale. *Age and Ageing*, 50(4): 1406–1411.

Trauma Audit and Research Network (2017). England and Wales. Major trauma in older people. Available at: https://aace.org.uk/wp-content/uploads/2017/04/Major-Trauma-in-Older-People-2017.pdf [accessed 27th September 2023].

Turner G (2014). Recognising frailty. British Geriatrics Society. Available at https://www.bgs.org.uk/resources/recognising-frailty [accessed 28th September 2023].

Woodford HJ (2022). *Essential Geriatrics* (4th edition). Oxon: CRC Press.

Xue QL (2011). The frailty syndrome: definition and natural history. *Clinics in Geriatric Medicine*, 27(1): 1–15.

Young RL, Smithard DG (2020). The Clinical Frailty Scale: do staff agree? *Geriatrics*, 5(2): 40.

Chapter 4

Long-Term Conditions

Tom Mallinson

Learning Points

By the end of this chapter, you will:

- Understand common long-term conditions that will help with holistic assessment of the patient
- Understand how long-term conditions are managed which will help with formulating management plans
- Understand that long-term conditions lead to older people needing to take multiple medications which can affect their susceptibility to other conditions or falls
- Understand that long-term conditions may mask acute presentations of illness or injury.

Case Study

Background: You are an ACP, on a rotational placement working in a primary care setting. Your next patient is 74-year-old Gayani.

Presenting Complaint: Atrial fibrillation (AFib).

History of Presenting Complaint: Gayani had an incidental finding of AFib when her pulse was checked last month by an ambulance crew following a non-injury fall: this has been confirmed on an ECG. She did not wish to attend hospital at the time as she had tripped and not been able to get herself back up.

Social History: She is active around the house and garden, looking after her five pet chickens and a dog.

Observations: She is otherwise well, with normal hepatorenal function and haematinics and a blood pressure of 166/73 mmHg.

CHAPTER 4   Long-Term Conditions

Initial Plan: Knowing that AFib increases the risk of future stroke, you are interested in finding out her bleeding risk profile so that you can discuss with your supervising GP whether she should be started on an anticoagulant. You are thinking either a DOAC or a coumarin.

Tool	Score	Bleeding Risk	Risk Group
ORBIT	0	Bleeds per 100 patient years 2.4	Low risk
HAS-BLED	2	Risk of major bleeding in 1 year with a DOAC 1.88–3.2%	Intermediate risk
ATRIA	1	Risk of bleeding in 1 year on warfarin 0.76%	Low risk

Gayani's CHA_2DS_2-VASc score is 2. This gives her a risk of having a stroke in the next year of 3.2% if she remains uncoagulated. The challenge of course is how best to convey this risk to Gayani, after all, 3.2% sounds like a small number, but for those patients who are unlucky enough to sustain a stroke it can be devastating. For most patients it is likely that the risks of anticoagulation are preferable to the risks of unrestricted thromboembolic events, however this should certainly be a shared decision made on an individual basis.

With this information, you speak to Gayani who would like to speak to her family before starting new medications. You agree and arrange a follow-up appointment.

Introduction

The management of long-term conditions (LTCs) is the bread and butter of primary and community care. Each older person we see, irrespective of clinical context, is increasingly likely to have an LTC that is being managed in primary care. Many of these patients will require home visits and therefore their LTCs will often be managed by paramedics, nurses and ACPs of all professional backgrounds. Understanding common LTCs is relevant for all clinicians working within a community setting, especially as many of these conditions form the multimorbidity background of many older adults when presenting with an acute illness or injury. Such management involves a balancing act of polypharmacy, medical complexity, diagnostic uncertainty and challenging clinical consultations. In many cases established best practice guidelines, written as they so often are by single-organ specialists, will be inappropriate for the patient in front of you and a Realistic Medicine approach will be required to provide the best care for your individual patient. In some cases a Realistic Medicine approach deviates from the strict confines of best practice, for example the patient and clinician may agree for less tight control of blood results, less frequent follow-up monitoring or a reduced burden in terms of investigations or treatments. Always ensure you are undertaking investigations for the benefit of the patient and not for your own clinical curiosity; for some older patients, invasive investigations may be unwanted, upsetting or lead to iatrogenic harm.

Asthma and Chronic Obstructive Pulmonary Disease (COPD)

In well controlled asthma, there is a risk that the patient will distance themselves from health services over time leading to poor adherence to prescribed medications and a lack of an up-to-date written asthma action plan. These are known risk factors for fatal asthma exacerbations (D'Amato et al., 2016).

Well controlled asthma should lead to no respiratory symptoms (cough, wheeze or breathlessness) for the majority of the time. There should be no sleep disruption due to the disorder, nor limitations to physical exertion. There should be an absence of acute asthma attacks and the patient should not be relying on frequent use of a beta-agonist (for example, salbutamol). Ideally the patient should also be free from troublesome side effects from their medications (Murtagh et al., 2018).

Primary care management of asthma seeks to give patients the knowledge and tools to manage their asthma as a lifelong condition. This requires effective coordination of the MDT and strategies to engage with patients in the long term (SIGN, 2019). The patient's knowledge of the disease means that in an acute episode they are experts in their own care and this is reflected in their own asthma action plan, an example of which is shown in Table 4.1.

Table 4.1 Personalised asthma action plan.

List of Asthma Triggers	To serve as a reminder or a checklist of exposures to consider if symptoms worsen.
Annual Asthma Review	A reminder to schedule this annually and what to bring: • This action plan • Peak flow meter/diary • Inhalers and other medications • Any questions for the clinician.
Exacerbation Triggers: **2–3 Action Points**	These can be triggered by symptoms or peak expiratory flow readings (PEFR). Suggested triggers could be: • PEFR <80% Best: Quadruple regular corticosteroid inhaler for two weeks. • PEFR <60% Best: Commence oral prednisolone and seek same-day medical advice. • PEFR <50% Best: Seek urgent medical advice.
Contact Details	This should include their GP practice, but also the contact details for the out of hours service in their area.
Treatment Regime	It is also useful to document the current daily treatment regime and how to modify this if symptoms worsen.

CHAPTER 4   Long-Term Conditions

Long-term management of asthma in the older population can be a challenge for a multitude of reasons. Diagnosis is more challenging in older people; delineating asthma and COPD can prove difficult and medical management is challenged by polypharmacy and multimorbidity. Asthma does, however, affect about 10% of the older adult population and patients in this group are around five times more likely to die as a result of their asthma than younger asthmatics (Bellia et al., 2007; Gonzalez-Diaz et al., 2019; Oraka et al., 2012). Asthma in older people is also often underdiagnosed and undertreated because of a number of factors, including increased patient tolerance for troublesome symptoms and clinicians accepting poor asthma control in this patient group (Melani, 2013). This appears to have a direct effect on the treatment older people receive for their asthma. They are less likely to be prescribed inhaled corticosteroids (Navaratnam et al., 2008) and are perhaps less likely to be taking them when they are prescribed (Gibson et al., 2010).

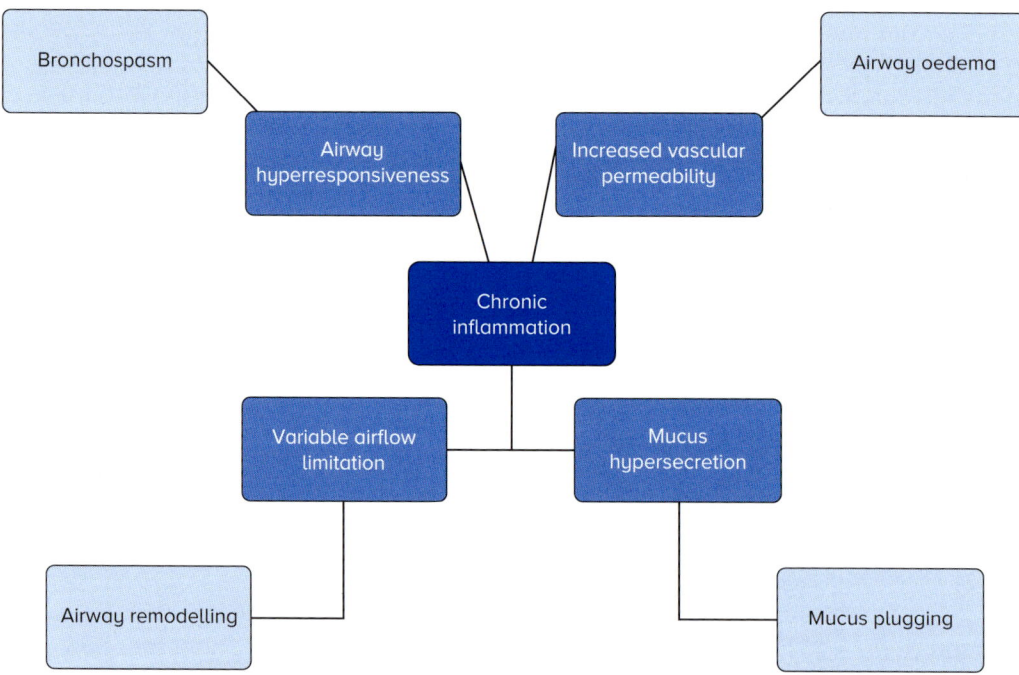

Figure 4.1   Sequalae of chronic airway inflammation.

In many cases it is difficult to accurately differentiate those with fully reversible airway disease (asthma) and those whose lungs have undergone remodelling due to long-standing lung disease (COPD) (see Figure 4.1).

In both asthma and COPD, courses of oral steroids or increasing inhaled steroids can be beneficial in reducing the inflammatory response and reducing symptoms. However, repeated use of corticosteroids in all patient groups, but especially older adults, creates the risk of a plethora of unwanted and potentially serious side effects (as set out in Box 4.1). The other medications used in both asthma and COPD also have the potential for significant unwanted side effects or drug interactions in relation to polypharmacy for older people (see Chapter 6: Polypharmacy and Medicines Review) (Newnham, 2001). Beta-agonists can cause palpitations (see 'Atrial fibrillation' later in this chapter), hypertension and hypokalaemia, while the theophyllines risk an array of side effects ranging from gastrointestinal upset to life-threatening dysrhythmias. The anticholinergic inhaled medications such as ipratropium are generally well tolerated but may exacerbate the anticholinergic burden experienced as a result of polypharmacy (see 'Anticholinergic burden' within Chapter 6: Polypharmacy and Medicines Review).

Box 4.1 Side Effects of Corticosteroid Treatment.

- Adrenal failure
- Cataracts
- Delirium/Psychosis
- Diabetes mellitus
- Ecchymosis
- Gastritis/Gastric ulceration
- Glaucoma
- Hypertension
- Hypoadrenalism
- Myopathy
- Osteoporosis

Heart Failure

The management of heart failure is medical (rather than surgical) for many patients and relies on carefully balanced polypharmacy to reduce both mortality and symptom burden (see Chapter 6: Polypharmacy and Medicines Review). A core aim in the management of heart failure with a reduced ejection fraction is the optimisation of blood pressure control. This is because hypertension causes an increase in the left ventricular afterload with associated increased peripheral vascular resistance. These raised pressures lead to remodelling of the left ventricle, compensatory ventricular hypertrophy and left atrial hypertrophy. This hypertrophy occurs to preserve cardiac output and delay decompensation. However, a hypertrophied heart is prone to developing stiffness, reduced contractility and diastolic dysfunction: when this happens sequelae such as pulmonary oedema occur as the patient decompensates.

While the exact target for blood pressure reduction is hotly debated, there is often a push from single-organ specialists to significantly reduce the blood pressure. This may be disadvantageous for the older person due to the consequences of hypotension, such as falls and the common sequelae of hip fractures and head injuries (see the comparative examples set out in Table 4.2). Finding the appropriate middle ground between avoiding both hypertension and hypotension is the realm of the primary and community care clinician, who must balance treatment for the patient's heart failure with any comorbidities. When searching for this middle ground, especially when titrating or switching medications, patients may experience unwanted sequelae and present to other services for their input.

CHAPTER 4 Long-Term Conditions

Table 4.2 Heart failure: comparative approaches.

Under-Treatment	Over-Treatment
Roberto is 75 years old and told his GP that he really did not want to be taking lots of tablets, as such he is only taking an angiotensin converting enzyme inhibitor (ACEi) and his blood pressure sits around 175/93. What are the benefits of this approach for the individual patient and for the wider health service?	Rhys is 78 years old. The local heart failure team have been very keen to lower their blood pressure with multiple antihypertensives. Their blood pressure now sits around 110/66 and the team are very happy with this. What are the benefits of this approach for the individual patient and for the wider health service?
What are the risks inherent with this treatment plan and how can they be both mitigated and discussed openly with the patient? Roberto benefits from a reduced tablet burden (compared to Rhys). He has expressed that this is important to him and therefore we are respecting his autonomy and ensuring a shared approach to treatment decisions. At a system level, there may be a cost saving factor related to fewer prescriptions and fewer check-ups to ensure his blood pressure is tightly controlled, however any increased disease burden or progression has the risk of requiring more intensive healthcare interventions later. Roberto is at risk of a faster disease progression with his heart failure and from the other pathologies linked to hypertension such as stroke or aortic aneurysm. These risks would need to be discussed with him to ensure he is making an informed decision.	What are the risks inherent with this treatment plan and how can they be both mitigated and discussed openly with the patient? We do not know how Rhys feels about the range of medications they are being asked to take and such intensive treatment may result in feelings of reassurance that everything is being done to optimise their health. Rhys is at risk of falls or collapses if their blood pressure runs too low to ensure cerebral perfusion at all times, including episodes of sudden exertion. Such a fall in an older patient poses a risk of significant traumatic injuries with associated morbidity and mortality. These are difficult risks to discuss as they involve the unpredictable incident of a fall. It is also unlikely that targeting a blood pressure lower than 130/80 has significant all-cause mortality benefit.

Aortic Stenosis

Aortic stenosis (AS), whether congenital or acquired, carries with it a significant burden in terms of morbidity and mortality. It occurs in around 3% of over 75s (Strange et al., 2021). Patients with mild or asymptomatic AS may not require any special monitoring but do need their consulting clinician to be on high alert for features of disease progression. Those with moderate disease may simply require the primary care team to ensure appropriate monitoring is in place and being adhered to, often with just routine follow-up to repeat echocardiograms. Once patients develop symptomatic AS it is unlikely any medical intervention will be of noticeable benefit, with surgical repair or replacement being the core treatment modality. Hypertension however is a key feature which can be modulated in primary and community care. Hypertension on a background of AS confers a higher risk of left ventricular remodelling and cardiovascular morbidity and mortality. For such patients, it is likely that the use of angiotensin converting enzyme inhibitors (ACEi) and angiotensin receptor blockers (ARBs) will facilitate a reduction in blood pressure while maintaining good left ventricular function (Sen et al., 2020).

Atrial Fibrillation

Atrial fibrillation (AFib) is disorganised electrical activity in the cardiac atria. It is the most common cardiac dysrhythmia worldwide (Lippi et al., 2021). It is characterised by inappropriate mechanical movement of the atria causing turbulent flow or stasis of blood, one of the elements of Virchow's Triad (see Figure 4.2), which in turn confers a risk of thromboembolism and subsequent stroke. Poorly controlled AFib also puts patients at risk of tachycardia induced cardiac remodelling resulting in heart failure and cardiomyopathy, cardiac ischaemia and a reduced exercise tolerance and lower quality of life (Lippi et al., 2021).

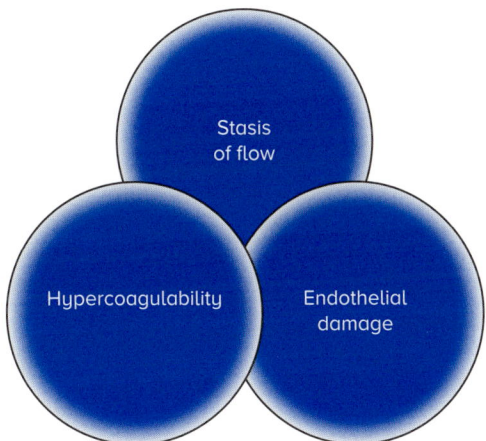

Figure 4.2 Virchow's Triad.

The are numerous causes of AFib (see Box 4.2 – Selected Causes of Atrial Fibrillation), so clinicians must be vigilant to spot patients with this condition. A manual pulse check can be a quick and easy indicator that AFib may be present. For any patient where an irregular pulse has been identified, an electrocardiogram (ECG) is required: this is usually initially in the form of a 12-lead ECG, although increasingly, point of care testing with handheld ECG machines is becoming more common. Some patients move into, and out of, the abnormal rhythm of AFib (paroxysmal AFib) and for these patients it may be more difficult to capture AFib on a single ECG, therefore ambulatory ECG monitoring will be more appropriate if this diagnosis is suspected.

CHAPTER 4 Long-Term Conditions

A 24-hour monitor is usually the best option, unless a patient describes intermittent symptoms over a longer period: in these cases an ambulatory ECG with an event recorder worn over a longer period may be more beneficial.

Box 4.2   Selected Causes of Atrial Fibrillation.

- Advanced age
- Alcohol
- Electrolyte disturbance
- Genetic predisposition
- Heart failure
- Hypertension
- Hyperthyroidism
- Ischaemic heart disease
- Medications (chemotherapy agents, bisphosphonates, NSAIDs and so on)
- Obesity
- Pneumonia
- Pyrexia
- Sleep apnoea
- Tobacco use

Once identified, steps should be taken to treat any underlying causes of the abnormal rhythm (that is, hyperthyroidism), but the AFib itself may also need to be addressed separately while treating a causative condition. Patients for whom AFib is caused by an underlying condition, where it is causing or worsening heart failure or where it is clearly a new onset of AFib, may be offered rhythm control, often electrical cardioversion. For others, the approach will likely be centred around rate control, usually with beta-blockers or with calcium channel blockade or digoxin.

Many cases of AFib can be appropriately managed in the community, but some require referral to secondary care (see Table 4.3). In the community most patients with AFib will receive rate control therapy, with beta-blockers (not sotalol). A rate limiting calcium channel blocker is the usual first line option. Digoxin may be used for sedentary patients with non-paroxysmal AFib. Diltiazem is also sometimes used concurrently to achieve adequate rate control. Amiodarone also has a place in initial rate control but should be avoided for long-term use.

Table 4.3   Referral for patients with atrial fibrillation.

Case Specifics	Referral Requirements
Severe symptoms of cardiovascular compromise	Immediate referral to hospital
Failure to rate control adequately	Refer within four weeks
Cardioversion or ablation is required	Refer to cardiology
Valvular disease is identified on ECG	Refer to cardiology
Other arrhythmogenic disorder identified (for example, Wolff–Parkinson–White, prolonged QT intervals)	Refer to cardiology

All patients with AFib (permanent or paroxysmal) should receive early assessment of their stroke and bleeding risks at diagnosis. This may be undertaken in primary care, in a dedicated AFib out-patient clinic or during a hospital admission. Stroke risk should be assessed using the CHA_2DS_2-VASc score and bleeding risk should be assessed using an appropriate tool: this is most likely to be the ORBIT score (Perry et al., 2021).

Several scoring systems do exist to allow the quantification of the risk that patients are exposed to when anticoagulated (HAS-BLED, ATRIA) (Fang et al., 2011; O'Brien et al., 2015; Pisters et al., 2010). These scores have each been validated slightly differently and one may be more appropriate for the patient in front of you than others, but ORBIT is generally recommended as the preferred tool (Perry et al., 2021).

The CHA_2DS_2-VASc is probably the most widely used score to predict risk of stroke and thromboembolic events for patients with AFib (Ntaios et al., 2013). It is only validated for non-valvular AFib. It does not include coronary artery disease or smoking status, which may be important additional risk factors, although this is unclear.

Depending on these scores and a discussion with the patient, an anticoagulant should be commenced. Choice of anticoagulant is nuanced but it is likely that one of the direct oral anticoagulants (DOACs) is preferrable to a coumarin (for example, warfarin) (Lee et al., 2021).

Diabetes

Long-term management of type 2 diabetes is far broader than establishing good glycaemic control and indeed overly tight goals for glycaemic control have been shown to result in worse outcomes. Even monitoring glycaemic control has some important potential pitfalls. For example, while HbA1c is an extremely useful test which does not require special actions from the patient, it cannot be used in a variety of situations. In cases where there may have been a rapid change in blood glucose levels, for example recent acute illness or concurrent steroid use, the result will be inaccurate due to the rapid rise in blood glucose. It is also not a reliable test in any situation where there is altered red cell lifespan, such as pregnancy, anaemia or any of the haemoglobinopathies (Beynon and Hillier, 2020; Kweka et al., 2019; Xu et al., 2021).

Management of diabetes is becoming an increasingly complex affair and is often delegated to a clinician with a specialist interest in this topic, be that one of the GPs or an allied health professional within the practice who can work with patients to formulate joint management plans. Managing patients with diabetes long-term involves a complex interplay of human factors and clinical medicine, with annual reviews being far more than a review of prescribed medication and diabetic foot health. Such longitudinal management can also be significantly disrupted when patients become increasingly frail or are admitted to care homes or nursing homes. Declines in physical activity and sudden changes in diet (for example, when meal selection is outsourced) may have drastic effects on blood sugar levels. This may require careful monitoring and adjustment of medications for a period.

Thyroid

The long-term management of disorders of the thyroid, especially hypothyroidism, is a key skill in primary care. In elders, the initial recognition of hypothyroidism may be challenging, as the early symptoms will likely masquerade as other common conditions prevalent in older people. These may include cold intolerance, weight gain, constipation, fatigue or low mood. Detecting clinical signs in the older population is equally challenging, as signs of hypothyroidism may include a relative bradycardia, pale or dry skin, evolving hoarseness or dysarthria and delayed relaxation on deep tendon reflex testing. As with younger patients, diagnosis is usually confirmed with the thyroid stimulating hormone (TSH) blood test. The first presentation within the older population may however be through other incidental abnormal findings on laboratory tests; all the following may indicate an undiagnosed hypothyroidism in the older patient: anaemia (hypochromic microcytic), hyponatraemia, hyperlipidaemia or a raised creatinine.

For older people, once a diagnosis has been confirmed, treatment with replacement thyroxine (usually in the form of levothyroxine) must be cautiously titrated. Iatrogenic hyperthyroidism can easily lead to significant tachydysrhythmias, anxiety or insomnia. It is likely that excess thyroxine will also exacerbate osteoporosis in the older population.

Stroke and Transient Ischaemic Attack

The immediate management of a suspected evolving stroke or transient ischaemic attack (TIA) follows the principle attributed to Dr Anna King that 'any sudden onset of central neurological signs or symptoms should be treated as a stroke until proven otherwise.' This involves promptly requesting an emergency ambulance and ensuring rapid access to neuroimaging. However, the long-term care of these patients is far more challenging.

Patients may present, for example, to primary or community care providers relaying a story of what sounds to have been a TIA which has now resolved. While such patients appear well in themselves (they must have achieved full symptom resolution to be defined as a TIA), a TIA is usually a warning of significant underlying pathology, most likely atherosclerotic disease. Therefore, these patients require urgent assessment in a specialist TIA clinic. As a primary or community care clinician, it may however be helpful to take a realistic overview of a patient's global health status before referral for further investigations; for example, a patient with a significant CFS score, or modified Rankin score, who would not be eligible for carotid endarterectomy perhaps should not undergo carotid doppler imaging.

Long-term management of patients living with stroke sequalae is, as with most chronic diseases, a multi-professional endeavour. Speech and language therapists, physiotherapists and occupational therapists will be key to facilitating a return to normality for many patients, even when they are left with neurological deficits. From the perspective of community care it will be vital to have a clear overview of the management plan put in place by the secondary care team and facilitate appropriate review and follow-up, especially in relation to antiplatelet regimens as most patients will be converted from aspirin to clopidogrel two weeks after their stroke. Blood pressure control is vital and usually changes to antihypertensives will be avoided in the acute phase, so titration of these may fall to primary care. The use of statins adds value for patients who have experienced an ischaemic stroke but may increase the risk of re-bleeding after haemorrhagic stroke. Expert advice should be sought for these patients.

Many patients will also experience psychological sequalae because of their stroke, with up to 15% of cases experiencing low mood so severe it causes suicidal ideation (Zhang et al., 2022). On assessment, we must be mindful of the whole patient and seek clues to identify the common significant mental health consequences of physical disease (see Chapter 5: Mental Health and Cognition for further information).

Parkinson's Disease

Parkinson's disease occurs because of the destruction of dopaminergic neurones in the brain. It is a progressive disease and brings with it a huge symptom burden for patients (Rogers et al., 2017). Many Parkinsonian symptoms can however be initially managed with non-pharmacological therapies and primary care clinicians may play a key role in facilitating access to these services, although increasingly specialist Parkinson's disease nurses are fulfilling this role. Early referral to therapy teams is indispensable; occupational therapy will allow assessment and input to facilitate ongoing independence, and physiotherapy input will also be especially useful for those with balance and other problematic motor symptoms. Speech and language therapy is beneficial for those with speech or swallowing issues. Early input from palliative medicine can also prove extremely positive for many patients, although others will be avoidant of this measure, so such referral decisions must be patient-centred in nature.

Further management can be divided for simplicity into mitigating motor symptoms and non-motor symptoms (Rogers et al., 2017). Motor symptoms are usually managed with a dopamine-mimetic (for example, levodopa) or other drugs which interact with dopamine receptors. While these medications do alleviate to some extent the symptomatology of movement disorders due to disease progression, they also expose the patient to several common side effects.

Non-motor symptoms are challenging to manage and may go undiagnosed for some time. They are worth specifically asking about during a consultation. Furthermore, many non-motor symptoms may be caused by the disease process itself or due to side effects from other medication being taken for Parkinson's disease. Because of this, medication changes for patients with Parkinson's disease

CHAPTER 4 Long-Term Conditions

need to be well thought through. Often the initiation of new medications or swapping from one drug to another is done with the support of, or by, secondary care Parkinson's specialists.

Iatrogenic Acute Kidney Injury

Several medications are well known for causing renal impairment through various mechanisms. The three main mechanisms are acute tubular injury, acute interstitial nephritis and crystalline nephropathy (see Table 4.4). Drugs can cause acute tubular injury through their innate toxicity. Patients who are dehydrated or hypotensive are at increased risk, as are those exposed to high doses or repeated exposure to nephrotoxic substances. Acute interstitial nephritis is an immune mediated form of renal injury, resulting from a T-cell mediated immune response and subsequent infiltration of the renal parenchyma by these cells leading to inflammation. Crystalline damage to the kidneys occurs, as its name suggests, through intratubular precipitation of drugs as crystals and a subsequent inflammatory response. Several other medications may lead to pseudo-acute kidney injury through a few varied mechanisms. Therefore, we must be constantly alert to polypharmacy and intercurrent illness which places a patient at increased risk of renal injury (see Chapter 6: Polypharmacy and Medicines Review).

Table 4.4 Mechanisms of iatrogenic acute kidney injury.

Acute Tubular Injury	Acute Interstitial Nephritis	Crystalline Nephropathies
Antibiotics	Antibiotics	Amoxicillin
Antivirals	Analgesics	Antivirals
Analgesics	Anticonvulsants	Ciprofloxacin
Bisphosphonates	Antivirals	Methotrexate
	Diuretics	

Osteoarthritis

Osteoarthritis (OA) is a common LTC in older people. It usually presents as worsening pain and limited functioning of a joint or joints with progressive impact on quality of life and ADLs (see Chapter 7: Activities of Daily Living). While OA was historically considered simple wear and tear of a joint, we now understand it to be a much more complex, and metabolically active, pathology (Mobasheri et al., 2017). A key feature of OA is the loss of the articular cartilages within synovial joints; however, many surrounding structures are also part of the disease process. Structural changes in surrounding tissues (subchondral bone, synovium, adjacent ligamental structures and adipose tissue) also adversely affect a joint's biomechanics and homeostatic pathways (Goldring and Goldring, 2016). It is perhaps best to consider OA as a pathology which initially manifests as abnormal joint tissue activity with subsequent anatomical and physiological changes resulting in functional impairment.

Long-term management of OA needs to be both holistic and multidisciplinary. In milder cases this may take the form of appropriate analgesia and facilitating access to either physiotherapy or sources of information for a patient to guide their own exercise regimen. In more advanced cases, a more complex interplay of professions may be required (see Figure 4.3).

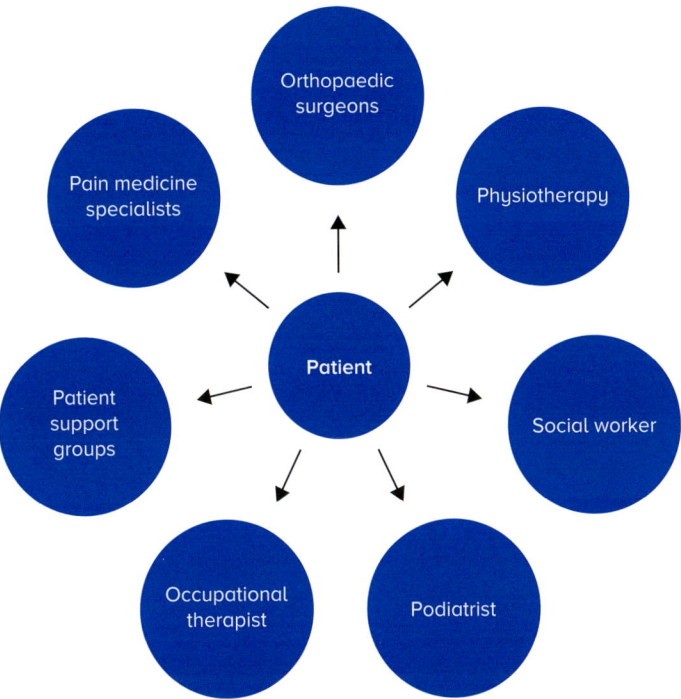

Figure 4.3 Multidisciplinary approach to osteoarthritis management.

Malignancy

Cancer treatment is complex and multifaceted, often requiring input from multiple specialists and professional groups. In established cancer, the role of the clinician in primary care may often be that of coordinator between these different specialists. However, the key intervention is more importantly the early recognition and referral of patients with suspected malignancy based on key signs and symptoms. These are often referred to in shorthand as two week wait (2ww) indicators, as they require a rapid referral for onward investigation utilising a two week wait pathway. To practice in primary and community care, you must be familiar with these and know where to seek clarification for the more unusual or rarely encountered presentations. The Scottish Referral Guidelines for Suspected Cancer are a good resource containing this information (NHS Scotland, 2019). An example of the referral criteria for head and neck cancers is shown in Box 4.3.

Box 4.3 Example Head and Neck Cancer Referral Guidance.

> Emergency referral
> - Stridor
>
> Urgent cancer referral
> - Persistent and unexplained head or neck lump for more than three weeks
> - Unexplained ulceration or swelling of the oral mucosa for more than three weeks
> - Unexplained red or mixed red/white patches on the oral mucosa for more than three weeks
> - Persistent hoarseness lasting more than three weeks
> - Persistent painful throat or odynophagia for more than three weeks

Chronic Pain

The management of pain is challenging for any clinician, but more than most, those working in primary care who are key for managing this as an LTC must balance the need for analgesia with the associated risks of addiction, sedation, delirium and falls in older people. There has been a recent initiative to reduce the prescribing of opioids (NICE, 2024), pregabalin and all antiepileptics, paracetamol, steroids, local anaesthetics and ketamine for patients with chronic primary pain. GPs have also been instructed not to utilise transcutaneous electrical nerve stimulation (TENS) or ultrasound for such patients (NICE, 2024), but acupuncture, exercise programmes and topical non-steroidal anti-inflammatory drugs (NSAIDs) or rubefacients are still being advocated.

This guidance significantly limits the options available to manage patients presenting with chronic pain and places greater emphasis than ever on the use of exercise programmes, physical activity and psychological therapies. This means that the care for older patients with chronic pain often becomes a matter of assisting them to navigate the various support groups available and in assisting with the coordination of a multidisciplinary pain team.

Conclusion

The management of LTCs for older people is challenging on many fronts. Diagnosis may be delayed or hampered by multimorbidity, polypharmacy or cognitive decline, with delays in diagnosis posing significant risks in terms of morbidity and mortality. Once a diagnosis has been made, the treatment of newly identified conditions is again complicated by the patient's other conditions and treatments. We must be on guard to avoid iatrogenic harm, especially through over-zealous interventions; as such, the maxim to 'start low and go slow' holds true for the majority of prescribing in the older population. Understanding the complexity that

LTCs bring to the assessment of older adults in the settings where paramedics and other community-based clinicians work is essential for effective clinical decision making. This involves a detailed consideration of the existing conditions and treatments already in place.

> **Questions**
>
> 1. Consider this chapter's content and apply what you have learnt to a recent patient or even a family member.
> 2. How would you change your approach to a patient with a similar presentation now, considering what you have read?
> 3. How do you make the link between LTCs and the various theories of ageing described in Chapter 1?

Further Resources

- Realistic medicine (2024). *Website*. Available at: https://realisticmedicine.scot/

References

Bellia V, et al. (2007). Asthma in the elderly: mortality rate and associated risk factors for mortality. *Chest*, 132(5): 1175–1182.

Beynon C, Hillier S (2020). Should HbA1C be used to screen pregnant women for undiagnosed diabetes in the first trimester? A review of the evidence. *Journal of Public Health*, 42(1): 132–140.

D'Amato G, et al. (2016). Asthma-related deaths. *Multidisciplinary Respiratory Medicine*, 11: 37.

Fang MC, et al. (2011). A new risk scheme to predict warfarin-associated hemorrhage: the ATRIA (Anticoagulation and Risk Factors in Atrial Fibrillation) study. *Journal of the American College of Cardiology*, 58(4): 395–401.

Gibson PG, McDonald VM, Marks GB (2010). Asthma in older adults. *The Lancet*, 376(9743): 803–813.

Goldring S, Goldring M (2016). Changes in the osteochondral unit during osteoarthritis: structure, function and cartilage-bone crosstalk. *Nature Reviews: Rheumatology*, 12: 632–644.

Gonzalez-Diaz SN, et al. (2019). Outcome measures to be considered on asthma in elderly. *Current Opinion in Allergy and Clinical Immunology*, 19(3): 209–215.

Kweka B, et al. (2019). Validity of HbA1c in diagnosing diabetes among people with sickle cell trait in Tanzania. *Blood*, 134(S1), 4852.

Lee JJ, et al. (2021). Meta-analysis of safety and efficacy of direct oral anticoagulants versus warfarin according to time in therapeutic range in atrial fibrillation. *The American Journal of Cardiology*, 140: 62–68.

Lippi G, Sanchis-Gomar F, Cervellin G (2021). Global epidemiology of atrial fibrillation: an increasing epidemic and public health challenge. *International Journal of Stroke*, 16(2): 217–221.

Melani AS (2013). Management of asthma in the elderly patient. *Clinical Interventions in Aging*, 8: 913–922.

Mobasheri A, et al. (2017). The role of metabolism in the pathogenesis of osteoarthritis. *Nature Reviews: Rheumatology*, 13: 302–311.

CHAPTER 4 Long-Term Conditions

Murtagh J, Rosenblatt J, Coleman JJ (2018). *John Murtagh's General Practice*. Sydney: McGraw-Hill Education Pty Limited.

National Institute for Health and Care Excellence (NICE) (2024). Chronic pain (NICE guideline NG193). Available at: https://www.nice.org.uk/guidance/ng193 [accessed 27th May 2024].

Navaratnam P, et al. (2008). Asthma pharmacotherapy prescribing in the ambulatory population of the United States: evidence of nonadherence to national guidelines and implications for elderly people. *The Journal of the American Geriatrics Society*, 56(7): 1312–1317.

Newnham DM (2001). Asthma medications and their potential adverse effects in the elderly. *Drug Safety*, 24(14): 1065–1080.

NHS Scotland (2019). Scottish referral guidelines for suspected cancer. Available at: https://www.cancerreferral.scot.nhs.uk [accessed 28th May 2024].

Ntaios G, et al. (2013). $CHADS_2$, CHA_2DS_2-VASc, and long-term stroke outcome in patients without atrial fibrillation. *Neurology*, 80(11): 1009–1017.

O'Brien EC, et al. (2015). The ORBIT bleeding score: a simple bedside score to assess bleeding risk in atrial fibrillation. *European Heart Journal*, 36(46): 3258–3264.

Oraka E, et al. (2012). Asthma prevalence among US elderly by age groups: age still matters. *Journal of Asthma*, 49: 593–599.

Perry M, et al. (2021). Atrial fibrillation: diagnosis and management – summary of NICE guidance. *British Medical Journal*, 373: n1150.

Pisters R, et al. (2010). A novel user-friendly score (HAS-BLED) to assess 1-year risk of major bleeding in patients with atrial fibrillation: the Euro Heart Survey. *Chest*, 138(5): 1093–1100.

Rogers G, et al. (2017). Parkinson's disease: summary of updated NICE guidance. *British Medical Journal*, 358: j1951.

Sen J, et al. (2020). Antihypertensive therapies in moderate or severe aortic stenosis: a systematic review and meta-analysis. *British Medical Journal Open*, 10(10): e036960.

SIGN (2019). SIGN 158: British guideline on the management of asthma. Available at: https://www.sign.ac.uk/media/1773/sign158-updated.pdf [accessed 14th October 2024].

Strange GA, et al. (2021). Uncovering the treatable burden of severe aortic stenosis in the UK. *Open Heart*, 9: e001783.

Xu Y, et al. (2021). Addressing shortfalls of laboratory HbA1c using a model that incorporates red cell lifespan. *Elife*, 10: e69456.

Zhang S, et al. (2022). Meta-analysis of risk factors associated with suicidal ideation after stroke. *Annals of General Psychiatry*, 21(1): 1–11.

Chapter 5

Mental Health and Cognition

Axel Laurell, Viveca Kirthisingha and Benjamin Underwood

Learning Points

By the end of this chapter, you will:

- Understand the presentation of dementia
- Understand the presentations of anxiety, depression, schizophrenia and deliberate self-harm
- Be able to formulate a plan for immediate management
- Know what further help might be appropriate for your patient.

Case Study

Background: You are a paramedic working in a GP practice and an electronic request comes in for a consultation with a relative who is worried about their mother being withdrawn and not eating for the last month.

Presenting Complaint: Change in behaviour and decreased oral intake.

History of Presenting Complaint: The patient's daughter tells you that her 78-year-old mother has been eating poorly since she fell and fractured her left humerus 3 months ago. She was reviewed by the fracture clinic and received intervention at home which included physiotherapy. Despite this support, her mobility has remained poor and she feels too tired and weak to move. She recently attended a clinic appointment with the orthopaedic team who did not find any medical reason for her weakness. She has told her daughter that the angel Saint Peter has been talking to her at night, telling her that her life is over and that it is time for her soul to be judged at the gates of heaven. The patient believes that her body gave up and died during her recent fall. Several times a day she comments on a lingering foul smell, which she likens to raw meat that has gone off. The patient believes that the smell comes from her organs slowly rotting from the inside. She has also contacted a local funeral director, enquiring about cremation so that her soul can finally be set free. Although the patient tells you that she is not worried about her mood, her

CHAPTER 5 Mental Health and Cognition

daughter says that she is often crying and appears anxious and hopeless. She feels that her continued existence is a burden on her family. She denies any thoughts of self-harm but asks you for help to dispose of her body, so that her rotting organs do not attract flies and other vermin into the house. The patient only eats when prompted to and she complains of always feeling nauseated. She is currently sleeping 5 hours per night, waking up at 04:00.

Past Medical History: Hypertension, recent humeral fracture and osteoarthritis. A six-month admission to a psychiatric hospital after the birth of her daughter when she received 'electrical treatment' but has not had any issues since.

Allergies: No known drug allergies

Drug History: Amlodipine (5 mg once daily), atorvastatin (20 mg at night), Adcal-D3 (1 tab twice daily), paracetamol (1 g as required).

Social History: The patient lives alone in a house without a package of care (POC). Prior to her fall she was independent with all ADLs. Her husband died six months ago and she has found it difficult to adjust to being alone at home. Prior to her fracture, the patient was an active volunteer for a local church which she visited several times per week. She has been a devout Christian for most of her life but has not attended any church services recently. She also has several friends in nearby villages which she used to see regularly for a knitting group and for long walks around the countryside. However, after her husband died she lost her motivation to attend these. Two of her daughters live nearby and she has several grandchildren that visit regularly. Since she fractured her humerus, she has been dependent on her daughters helping her with shopping, cooking and cleaning. The patient is a non-smoker and rarely drinks alcohol.

Assessment

- **GCS score:** 15
- **Heart rate:** 60 bpm
- **Blood pressure:** 140/80 mmHg
- **Respiratory rate:** 16 breaths per minute
- **Oxygen saturations:** 99% on air
- **Temperature:** 36.8°C
- **Pupils:** Equal and reactive
- **NEWS2 score:** 0
- **Mood:** Appears objectively low
- **CFS Score:** 3 (prior to current illness)
- **4AT Delirium score:** 0

Examination

The patient is slightly underweight. She is sitting in a wheelchair. Her daughter helped her to wash earlier and she is wearing clean and appropriate clothes. The house is also clean. Her eye contact is good, but she speaks minimally throughout the assessment and you get most information from speaking to her daughter. She repeatedly apologises to you for the foul smell as she is convinced that she 'stinks' and is 'rotting'. Objectively, you are not able to detect any foul smell. On auscultation, her chest is clear and heart sounds are normal. The abdomen is soft and non-tender and neurological examination is normal. She is oriented to time, place and person.

Holistic Assessment

The patient's daughter is worried that her mum has an undiagnosed physical illness or that she is developing dementia. She feels that her mum has been going downhill since her husband's death and that she has been increasingly isolating herself from her friends and family. She spends most of her time in bed and the family are struggling to motivate her to have a shower or to leave the house. The daughter is particularly worried that her mum has been losing weight and that she keeps talking about cremation and her funeral. Her daughter feels that the family is no longer able to provide enough support at home and that she needs to be transferred to a hospital or a care home. The patient and daughter together complete the Patient Health Questionnaire (PHQ)-9 form, a screening test for depression, and she scores 23/27.

Initial Impression: Severe depressive episode with psychotic symptoms.

Initial Plan:

- Arrange blood tests including FBC, U&E, liver function tests, thyroid function tests (TFTs), bone profile, vitamin B12, folate and CRP to exclude any underlying physical illness, nutritional status and dehydration causing a delirium. If the results indicate an acute or life-threatening physical illness, the patient may need admission to a general hospital for medical assessment and treatment.

- Due to the risks described and the likelihood of a significant mental illness, a psychiatric opinion should be quickly sourced, possibly via a psychiatric crisis team. They may carry out a full psychiatric assessment to determine whether the patient meets the threshold for psychiatric in-patient admission and facilitate assessment under the Mental Health Act if that is required. Be aware that the type of assessment and support that psychiatric services can offer may vary depending on local provision. If the patient's level of risk does not meet the threshold for psychiatric in-patient admission, the crisis team can often organise regular reviews at home. They will assess the patient's mental and physical health and implement a biopsychosocial approach to treatment which is likely to include medication, psychological and behavioural approaches. In this case there are strong suggestions in the history and examination of psychotic features, including possible delusions and hallucinations. Psychiatric services may organise prescription of antidepressant or antipsychotic medication and can advise on onward referral to social and psychological services for support. If the person remains in the community, then the case would also benefit from discussion at the GP practice's weekly MDT meeting to cover physical, mental and social needs.

CHAPTER 5 Mental Health and Cognition

Introduction

Older people can experience the full range of mental disorders of adult life. In addition, older people are more likely to develop organic brain disorders that underlie dementia, including Alzheimer's disease, vascular dementia and Parkinson's disease (van der Flier and Scheltens, 2005). For these reasons, a grasp of the common mental disorders, their presentation, immediate management and the services that can provide help is essential when dealing with older people. Most psychiatric services are based in the community in the UK and extensive help in and out of hours is available. How to access these services may vary by geographical location, so knowing how to do so prior to needing them is important. This will be outlined in local service guidelines, policies, protocols and pathways.

Dementia

Dementia is a syndrome which causes a progressive decline in cognitive function. The prevalence of dementia doubles every 5 years after the age of 65 and thus affects around a third of people over the age of 90 (van der Flier and Scheltens, 2005). Alzheimer's disease is the most common form of dementia and occurs due to the toxic accumulation of misfolded proteins, causing progressive neuronal death (Scheltens et al., 2021). Short-term memory is usually affected first, but the impairment eventually spreads to affect other brain functions. The median survival is around five years (Scheltens et al., 2021). Vascular dementia is the second most common presentation of dementia and is caused by an impairment of the blood vessels that supply the brain (O'Brien and Thomas, 2015). The presentation of vascular dementia is more varied than that of Alzheimer's disease and depends on the area of the brain that is predominantly affected. There are also many other causes of dementia such as dementia with Lewy bodies, frontotemporal dementia and other neurodegenerative diseases, all of which have their own unique presentations (van der Flier and Scheltens, 2005). In clinical practice people often present with a mix of symptoms and in the very old the corresponding pathology is usually mixed too. It can be difficult to determine a single cause of a person's dementia and treatment is usually based on the most likely pathology.

Assessment

Any person presenting with a memory complaint requires a thorough assessment. Although healthy ageing is associated with a gradual reduction in memory, selective attention and executive function, these impairments are mild and do not usually affect independent living (Irwin et al., 2018). It is important to clarify whether the patient's symptoms started suddenly, which could indicate delirium or possibly a vascular origin, or whether they have been gradually worsening, which is more consistent with Alzheimer's disease or other neurodegenerative diseases (Elahi and Miller, 2017). A person with sudden onset memory problems should always be urgently investigated to exclude serious physical causes. A collateral history from a family member is essential to exploring the impact on ADLs. A CFS score can assist with identifying those who have had an acute change by assessing their baseline (two weeks ago) with how they present today (Rockwood et al., 2005). Other conditions, such as depression and delirium, as well as side effects of psychotropic medications, opioids, anticholinergics and polypharmacy, need to be excluded as they may mimic the symptoms of dementia. A physical examination is important to assess for signs of neurological diseases such as Parkinson's disease or previous strokes. A blood screen should be completed to rule out vitamin deficiencies, electrolyte disturbances and thyroid disease as these can also affect cognition. If dementia is clinically suspected, a memory screening test should be performed to objectively measure and characterise the areas of deficiency. The general practitioner assessment of cognition (GPCOG) is a screening test which is free and easy to administer. It has a high sensitivity and specificity for diagnosing dementia (Tsoi et al., 2015). It produces a score based on information from both the person and a close informant, indicating whether further investigations for a cognitive impairment are required.

Key Considerations

People living with dementia are at risk if they lose the ability to carry out ADLs. Consider whether the person needs a referral to social care or to sources of support such as the Alzheimer's Society or other local services (see Chapter 11: Social Care and Chapter 12: Safeguarding).

Legal or Ethical Considerations

People can appoint a Lasting Power of Attorney under the Mental Capacity Act 2005. This is usually a family member who is given the authority to make decisions about the person's welfare and/or finances if the person loses the mental capacity to make these decisions.

People who lack capacity to make decisions about their care can be treated in their best interests (Mental Capacity Act 2005). Box 5.1 outlines the principles of the Mental Capacity Act along with the two-stage test of capacity which must be met to determine that the person lacks capacity. This act governs the treatment of people who lack capacity in England and Wales. Similar acts exist in Scotland (Adults with Incapacity (Scotland) Act 2000) and in Northern Ireland (Mental Capacity Act (Northern Ireland) 2016). Whereas the assessment of capacity is similar, the practical application varies depending on which act is used. Readers should familiarise themselves with the particular act relevant to the nation in which they practice.

Capacity is specific to each decision. For example, a person may have the capacity to make basic decisions about their care but lack the capacity to decide on more complex interventions, like surgery. Capacity can also fluctuate over time and at the point of assessment every effort needs to be made to maximise capacity. Simple interventions might include helping the person to remain calm, making sure they have working hearing aids and glasses and ensuring they have familiar people around them for support. The person needs to demonstrate that they can understand the information, weigh-up the benefits and risks and retain this long enough to be able to communicate their reasoning and decision. It is important to document the decision the person is being asked to make and the reasons for suspecting that the person lacks capacity. Documentation should include the underlying disorder of the brain or

CHAPTER 5 Mental Health and Cognition

mind and how this impairs the person's ability to understand, recall and weigh-up the risks and to communicate their views (see Box 5.1 below). If a person is found to lack capacity, then documentation must include the decision that the care professional has made and why this is felt to be in the person's best interests.

Box 5.1 Principles of the Mental Capacity Act.

The Principles of the Mental Capacity Act 2005

1. A person must be assumed to have capacity unless it is established that they lack capacity.
2. A person is not to be treated as unable to make a decision unless all practicable steps to help them to do so have been taken without success.
3. A person is not to be treated as unable to make a decision merely because they make an unwise decision.
4. An act done, or decision made, under this Act for or on behalf of a person who lacks capacity must be done, or made, in their best interests.
5. Before the act is done, or the decision is made, regard must be had to whether the purpose for which it is needed can be as effectively achieved in a way that is less restrictive of the person's rights and freedom of action.

Two-Stage Test of Capacity

1. Does the person have an impairment of, or a disturbance in the functioning of, their mind or brain?
2. Does the impairment or disturbance mean that the person is unable to make a specific decision when they need to?

A person lacks capacity to make a decision for themselves if they are unable:

- To **understand** the information relevant to the decision
- To **retain** that information for long enough to make the decision
- To **use or weigh-up** that information as part of the process of making the decision
- To **communicate** their decision.

Decisions about the care of people who lack capacity can be challenging and senior clinical advice should be sought where required.

Management

People who get referred to the memory clinic will have the history of their memory problems revisited and will have more extensive cognitive tests performed. Most people will subsequently have brain imaging to support and subtype the diagnosis. Treatment should be focussed on improving quality of life and supporting the person to live independently. There are a range of assistive technologies, including video monitoring, GPS (global positioning system) trackers and alarms, which can help people living with dementia and their caregivers to mitigate the risk of falls and wandering behaviours (Pappadà et al., 2021). There are also several smartphone apps which can assist with daily tasks, medication compliance and communication with family members. Assistive technology, as well as fire-resistant equipment, may reduce the risk of people with dementia experiencing accidental fires (Heward and Kelly, 2020). Caregivers should contact the local fire service to book a home visit for a safety check. People who are diagnosed with Alzheimer's disease will be offered an anticholinesterase inhibitor or memantine, both of which are associated with a modest improvement in cognition (Birks, 2006). They may also be offered medications for symptomatic treatment of agitation, low mood or psychosis (Livingston et al., 2017). Family members should be signposted to organisations such as the Alzheimer's Society which provides information and carer support.

Management of an Acute Medical Illness in Patients Diagnosed with Dementia

Acute care providers often face making difficult decisions when assessing people with dementia who have an acute medical illness. Although admission may be unavoidable, it is important to always consider community management as an option. One large, multicentre study found that the use of hospital at home services was associated with a reduced proportion of people with dementia moving to residential care, reduced rates of delirium and reduced costs for the healthcare service (Shepperd et al., 2022). There was no difference in mortality between those who were admitted and those who were managed in the community. This suggests that community management can be safe and can lead to better outcomes for people with dementia. If a decision is made to manage a person in the community, it is important to ensure that adequate follow-up is in place. It is not realistic for an ambulance crew to communicate with all the parties involved, so it is important to liaise with a member of the community services who can coordinate the care. This may be the GP or other senior members of the community services, such as a community matron or an ACP.

Delirium

Delirium is covered within Chapter 3: Frailty. There are some specific points included to help differentiate between acute and long-term impaired cognition. Delirium is an acute confusional state which occurs secondary to an acute medical illness (Adamis et al., 2007). It commonly occurs in people with dementia, sometimes in response to minor illnesses (Inouye et al., 2014). In older adults there is usually more than one cause and the confusion can persist for a long time after the initial trigger has resolved. Unlike most dementias, delirium has a sudden onset, impairs attention, is associated with sleep/wake disturbance and is often reversible. Delirium needs to be actively recognised, investigated and treated (Robertson, 2022).

Anxiety and Depression

Major depressive disorder affects up to 5% of older people (Fiske et al., 2009), with women, people with chronic health conditions, people with dementia and those living in deprived areas being at greater risk (McDougall et al., 2007). Many people have a history of depressive episodes earlier in life which may be triggered in later life by stressful life events, loss of social roles or a loss of functional independence (Fiske et al., 2009). There is also evidence suggesting that depression can be a risk factor for future cognitive decline as well as an early sign of a person developing dementia (Dafsari and Jessen, 2020). Consequently, it is important to take a comprehensive history from both the person and their family to get an accurate diagnosis.

Anxiety disorders often overlap with depression and affect around 10% of older adults (Wolitzky-Taylor et al., 2010). Most anxiety disorders usually present initially in young adulthood, but symptoms can be unmasked in older age due to stressful events (for example, a fall) or the loss of stabilising life factors (for example, the loss of a spouse).

Assessing Depression

Older people may underplay low mood and sadness, causing the diagnosis to be missed. They may present with excessive worrying over their physical health or with medically unexplained symptoms. People with depression often have reduced motivation, energy and pleasure from activities that they used to enjoy. It is helpful to get an idea of what their interests were prior to their illness. Older people with depression may also display psychotic symptoms more frequently than younger people (Gournellis et al., 2014). It is important to further explore any 'odd' ideas and beliefs. Delusions are often nihilistic in nature with themes of hopelessness and guilt and people can sometimes be convinced that they are dying or rotting ('Cotard's syndrome', Debruyne et al., 2009). People with psychotic depression can also experience auditory hallucinations, which typically manifest as voices making derogatory remarks or suggesting the person harm themselves. In contrast, visual hallucinations are uncommon and should prompt investigations for another diagnosis.

Assessing Anxiety Disorders

People with anxiety disorders experience both psychiatric symptoms (for example, fear and worrying) and physical symptoms (for example, palpitations, nausea and sweating) which significantly affects their daily functioning and can be challenging to differentiate from an organic illness. Common examples of anxiety disorders include specific phobia (for example, a fear of spiders), agoraphobia (that is, fear of leaving home) and social anxiety disorder (fear of speaking in front of others). When the anxiety occurs in multiple contexts it is classified as 'generalised anxiety disorder'. If the symptoms of fear and physical discomfort are sudden and intense it is 'panic disorder'. Other illnesses, such as post-traumatic stress disorder (PTSD), obsessive-compulsive disorder (OCD) and eating disorders also sit on the spectrum of anxiety disorders but are outside of the scope of this chapter.

Key Considerations

It is important to ask people with low mood or anxiety whether they have self-harmed and if they have any thoughts of suicide. Deliberate self-harm, even if it appears to be trivial, should not be dismissed as people over 65 years who self-harm go on to complete suicide at a higher rate than younger people who self-harm (Troya et al.,

2019). Furthermore, self-harm may not correlate with the severity of depression and everyone who presents in this way should receive a full psychosocial assessment. It is also important to consider the person's nutritional and hydration status at assessment through careful history taking, examination and possibly blood tests. Potential consequences of immobility and poor nutrition such as pressure ulcers, venous embolism or infection needs to be recognised and treated. People that have inadequate oral intake may need transfer to hospital for intravenous or subcutaneous fluids. In severe illness, electroconvulsive therapy (ECT) may also be considered which can lead to an improvement of depressive symptoms more rapidly than medications. Despite sometimes being portrayed as a controversial treatment in mainstream media, ECT is a widely used, effective and often lifesaving treatment for people with severe depression (Deng et al., 2024). It is a safe procedure with risks similar to other procedures requiring a general anaesthetic. Short-term memory impairment is a recognised side effect of ECT, but is also a feature of the underlying depression (Deng et al., 2024).

Legal or Ethical Considerations

People with severe depression who are at high risk to themselves may refuse admission to a mental health or general hospital for treatment and this would be an indication to consider an urgent Mental Health Act assessment following locally agreed referral or escalation pathways. This is governed by the Mental Health Act 1983 (amended 2007) in England and Wales, the Mental Health (Care and Treatment) (Scotland) Act 2003 in Scotland and the Mental Health (Northern Ireland) Order 1986. The powers and practical application vary depending on which act is relevant in the local area. Where possible, clinicians who are providing care on scene should request senior clinical advice to help safety-net people who may not wish to attend hospital, to enable access to appropriate pathways of care within the community.

Management

Treatment of anxiety and depression in older adults should be tailored around the needs of the individual. Both pharmacological and non-pharmacological measures should be considered (Fiske et al., 2009). A variety of psychological therapies, such as cognitive behavioural therapy (CBT), may be beneficial, although these can take time to access. It is also important to consider certain social issues when addressing some of the triggers and in order to prevent relapse. For example, good housing, regular activities and exercise and preventing social isolation can be very important for the individual (see Box 5.2). Treatment of physical illnesses should be optimised and mobility, eyesight and hearing should be reviewed. Many people require treatment with antidepressants, which are effective for both anxiety and depression. There are a variety of antidepressants available and their different side-effect profiles should be tailored to suit the individual. Antipsychotic medications can be used in addition to antidepressants if psychotic symptoms such as delusions or hallucinations are present. However, antipsychotics can be associated with significant side effects, therefore such prescribing is usually led by psychiatrists (NHSE, 2022). The prognosis is generally good, although it can take several weeks before an effect is apparent (Steinert et al., 2014).

CHAPTER 5 Mental Health and Cognition

Box 5.2 Loneliness and Social Isolation.

> Loneliness and social isolation are recognised as concepts that contribute to increased mortality in older people (Holt-Lunstad et al., 2015). Age UK (2018) describe the differences between the two terms. People can be isolated (alone), but not feel lonely. People can be surrounded by other people, yet still feel lonely. They further state that loneliness is a subjective feeling whereas social isolation is an objective measure of the number of contacts people have. Social isolation and loneliness are associated with depressive symptoms (Ge et al. 2017).

Deliberate Self-Harm

Deliberate self-harm is common across the lifespan and is a significant risk factor for completed suicide (Bachmann, 2018). It is more common in women and those with long-term psychiatric or physical health problems. Although deliberate self-harm appears to be less prevalent in older people, it is more frequently associated with repeated self-harm and completed suicide (Troya et al., 2019). For this reason, older adults who self-harm should always receive a thorough assessment to evaluate the triggers of the episode. Self-poisoning is the most common method in older adults, possibly due to increased access to medications, with many people also having suicidal intent (Troya et al., 2019). The reasons for self-harming can be complex. People can describe that they feel that their life has become meaningless and that they are struggling to cope with the loss of control and independence associated with ageing (Wand et al., 2018). Self-harming may be a way of taking back control of a situation that they feel is hopeless. Adverse life events, such as the loss of loved ones, an episode of ill health or the loss of social support can also be important triggers (Wand et al., 2018).

Assessment

Emergency care providers are commonly called to see people who have self-harmed. The assessment can be complex, especially if the person is distressed and refusing to provide any history or personal details. It is important to estimate the risk to physical health. In the case of an overdose, the type of substance and the quantity that the person has taken should be clarified. Every older person who has self-harmed should be properly assessed and monitored, even if the injury appears trivial. Transfer to ED should be prompt as some treatments, such as acetylcysteine, which is used for paracetamol overdose, have a specific timeframe for effectiveness (Ferner et al., 2011).

Legal or Ethical Considerations

During the initial phase of the incident, the attending clinician needs to assess the person's capacity using the principles of the Mental Capacity Act (Box 5.1). This is particularly important for individuals who refuse transport to an ED. However, every case is individual and each person and their circumstances must be assessed in order to provide the most appropriate care. Organisations should have access to senior clinicians who can support decision making (either on scene or remotely) within the legal frameworks available.

There might be legitimate concerns regarding the person's capacity to refuse transfer to hospital, particularly if they have consumed medication or alcohol, or are distressed. Taking the time to calm the situation and adjusting communication methods may be helpful. Joint Royal College Ambulance Liaison Committee (JRCALC) guidelines provide useful information for the assessment and decision making in such challenging situations (JRCALC and AACE, 2019). In practice, it may be that a person in distress who has self-harmed lacks capacity to make the decision about attending ED. If conveyance is felt to be in the best interests of a person lacking capacity to make decisions about their care, then the Mental Capacity Act might be appropriate legislation under which to provide treatment. In difficult situations where people refuse care, further advice should be urgently sought from senior staff and the wider health system.

Management

Management of individuals who have taken an overdose should be directed by the type and quantity of substance that has been used. Toxbase is an online toxicology database which is useful for guiding medical management. The National Poisons Information Centre also has a 24-hour phone line for emergency care providers which can be used to obtain urgent advice (see Further Resources at the end of the chapter). These sources can give advice on both the immediate treatments, like activated charcoal or naloxone, and the need for physical health monitoring. All people who have self-harmed should be referred to the local mental health service for a biopsychosocial assessment while in ED. The outcome of the assessment depends on the precipitants and the intent underlying the episode of self-harm. The person may be discharged home with support from the local crisis team, community mental health team or other services, or less commonly they may be admitted to a psychiatric hospital.

Schizophrenia

Schizophrenia is a chronic psychotic mental disorder which affects around 0.5% of older people (Cohen et al., 2015). It has a bimodal presentation with peaks in young adulthood and again in later life (Jauhar et al., 2022). Although the causes are poorly understood it has a high genetic heritability and appears related to abnormal neurodevelopment (McCutcheon et al., 2020). However, environmental risk factors such as urban living, substance misuse and childhood trauma are also important. Schizophrenia is noted as 'very late onset' if it presents for the first time after age 60. This late presentation is more common in women who often have long histories of being somewhat reclusive with limited family and social networks (Cohen et al., 2015). In addition, they often live with sensory impairment.

Signs, Symptoms and Assessment

The positive symptoms of schizophrenia include delusions, hallucinations and thought disorder which might manifest as speech that is hard to follow (Jauhar et al., 2022). The term 'positive' refers to symptoms that represent an addition of behaviours or experiences that are not typically present in healthy individuals. For instance, people with schizophrenia may feel persecuted and develop elaborate delusions that people wish them harm. In contrast, negative symptoms generally develop later in the illness (McCutcheon et al., 2020). They include social withdrawal, lack of pleasure, apathy, poor motivation and often manifest as reduced speech output, self-neglect and decreased expression of emotion. 'Negative' symptoms reflect a decrease in the abilities and characteristics that were once present. Older people with schizophrenia tend to have less disorganised speech than younger people (Cohen et al., 2015). They also have a higher degree of atypical visual, olfactory or tactile hallucinations, including 'partition delusions' where the assumed malign influence of others can be directed through walls. Cognitive impairment is a common feature of older people with schizophrenia and all patients will require a thorough assessment and follow-up to differentiate their symptoms from dementia (Suen et al., 2019).

Risks to Patient Safety

The risks surrounding the person need to be carefully assessed. Risks may include possible self-neglect, thoughts of direct harm to themselves or harm to those they perceive as persecuting them. Other risks may be less obvious, for example putting their tenancy in jeopardy through their behaviour or being vulnerable to exploitation by others (see Chapter 12: Safeguarding).

Legal or Ethical Concerns

People who require in-patient care may decline admission to hospital. Consideration would then have to be given as to the legal framework required to appropriately manage risk and deliver care. One option is to organise a Mental Health Act assessment which requires the presence of two doctors and an approved mental health practitioner (AMHP) (Mental Health Act, 1983). Advice on this can be sought via the duty AMHP service, emergency psychiatric services or locally agreed pathways for referral or escalation. Mental health law differs in Scotland and Northern Ireland and clinicians working in these areas should familiarise themselves with the local implementation of the act.

Management

People with schizophrenia should be managed using a multidisciplinary biopsychosocial approach. Most people will be offered antipsychotic treatment, which has been shown to be effective in a randomised controlled trial in older people (Howard et al., 2018), and receive long-term follow-up by the community mental health team. Psychological therapy including social skills training, cognitive training and CBT can also be helpful in improving executive functioning and improving community integration (Cohen et al., 2015). Overall, people with schizophrenia have a reduced life expectancy and are more likely to require long-term supportive and general medical care compared with the general population (Cohen et al., 2015).

Conclusion

Mental illness and cognitive decline are common in older people who often present with a complex mix of physical and mental health problems, polypharmacy and sensory impairment making the assessment more challenging. This chapter has illustrated some of the common presentations of mental illness in old age, focusing on the practical management in a non-specialist setting. Acute care providers must often decide where their patient is best managed – in the community or in a medical or psychiatric hospital – and how that care is accessed. When making these judgements, confidence in assessing mental capacity and how to screen for delirium and dementia are important. It is most helpful to be aware what community services are available locally and how to contact them prior to needing to do so.

> **Questions**
>
> 1. Consider this chapter's content and apply what you have learnt to a recent patient or event.
> 2. How would you change your approach to an older person with a mental health presentation, considering what you have read?
> 3. How would you adjust your communication to ensure a mental capacity assessment is valid?

Further Resources

- Age UK (n.d.). *Support with health, well-being, and finances for older people.* Available at: https://www.ageuk.org.uk
- Alzheimer's Society (n.d.). *Delirium symptoms, diagnosis and treatment.* Available at: https://www.alzheimers.org.uk/get-support/daily-living/delirium
- Alzheimer's Society (n.d.). *Dementia information and support.* Available at: https://www.alzheimers.org.uk
- Mind (n.d.). *Mental health support services.* Available at: https://www.mind.org.uk
- National Poisons Information Service (n.d.). *Poisons information services.* Available at: https://www.npis.org
- Toxbase (n.d.). *The primary clinical toxicology database of the National Poisons Information Service.* Available at: https://www.toxbase.org
- YouTube (2016). *Delirium Awareness Video.* Available at: https://www.youtube.com/watch?v=BPfZgBmcQB8
- People experiencing a mental health crisis can contact NHS 111, their general practitioner, or their local mental health service for support. Several free helplines are available for anyone experiencing a mental health crisis or thoughts about self-harming:
  - Samaritans – 116 123
  - Campaign Against Living Miserably (CALM) – 0800 58 58 58 (5 pm to midnight)
  - SOS Silence of Suicide – 0300 102 0505 (4 pm to midnight)

CHAPTER 5   Mental Health and Cognition

References

Adamis D, et al. (2007). A brief review of the history of delirium as a mental disorder. *History of Psychiatry*, 18(4): 459–469.

Adults with Incapacity (Scotland) Act (2000). Available at: https://www.legislation.gov.uk/asp/2000/4/contents [accessed 17th May 2024].

Age UK (2018). All the lonely people: loneliness in later life. Available at: https://www.ageuk.org.uk/globalassets/age-uk/documents/reports-and-publications/reports-and-briefings/loneliness/loneliness-report.pdf [accessed 17th May 2024].

Bachmann S (2018). Epidemiology of suicide and the psychiatric perspective. *International Journal of Environmental Research and Public Health*, 15(7): 1425.

Birks JS (2006). Cholinesterase inhibitors for Alzheimer's disease. *Cochrane Database of Systematic Reviews*, 1: CD005593.

Cohen CI, Meesters PD, Zhao J (2015). New perspectives on schizophrenia in later life: implications for treatment, policy, and research. *The Lancet Psychiatry*, 2(4): 340–350.

Dafsari FS, Jessen F (2020). Depression – an underrecognized target for prevention of dementia in Alzheimer's disease. *Translational Psychiatry*, 10(1): 1–13.

Debruyne H, et al. (2009). Cotard's syndrome: a review. *Current Psychiatry Reports*, 11(3): 197–202.

Deng Z-D, et al. (2024). How electroconvulsive therapy works in the treatment of depression: is it the seizure, the electricity, or both? *Neuropsychopharmacology*, 49(1): 150–162.

Elahi FM, Miller BL (2017). A clinicopathological approach to the diagnosis of dementia. *Nature Reviews Neurology*, 13(8): 457–476.

Ferner RE, Dear JW, Bateman DN (2011). Management of paracetamol poisoning. *British Medical Journal*, 342: d2218.

Fiske A, Wetherell JL, Gatz M (2009). Depression in older adults. *Annual Review of Clinical Psychology*, 5: 363–389.

Ge L, et al. (2017). Social isolation, loneliness and their relationships with depressive symptoms: a population-based study. *PLoS One*, 12(8): e0182145.

Gournellis R, Oulis P, Howard R (2014). Psychotic major depression in older people: a systematic review. *International Journal of Geriatric Psychiatry*, 29(8): 784–796.

Heward M, Kelly F (2020). Research and education to understand fire risks associated with dementia: a collaborative case study (innovative practice). *Dementia*, 19(7): 2477–2483.

Holt-Lunstad J, et al. (2015). Loneliness and social isolation as risk factors for mortality: a meta-analytic review. *Perspectives on Psychological Science*, 10(2): 227–337.

Howard R, et al. (2018). Antipsychotic treatment of very late-onset schizophrenia-like psychosis (ATLAS): a randomised, controlled, double-blind trial. *The Lancet Psychiatry*, 5(7): 553–563.

Inouye SK, Westendorp RG, Saczynski JS (2014). Delirium in elderly people. *The Lancet*, 383(9920): 911–922.

Irwin K, et al. (2018). Healthy aging and dementia: two roads diverging in midlife? *Frontiers in Aging Neuroscience*, 10: 275.

Jauhar S, Johnstone M, McKenna PJ (2022). Schizophrenia. *The Lancet*, 399(10323): 473–486.

Joint Royal College Ambulance Liaison Committee (JRCALC) and Association of Ambulance Chief Executives (AACE) (2024). JRCALC clinical guidelines. Version iOS 2.4(3). Bridgwater: Class Publishing. Available at: https://jrcalcplus.co.uk [accessed 1st April 2024].

Livingston G, et al. (2017). Dementia prevention, intervention, and care. *The Lancet*, 390(10113): 2673–2734.

McCutcheon RA, Reis Marques T, Howes OD (2020). Schizophrenia – an overview. *JAMA Psychiatry*, 77(2): 201–210.

References

McDougall FA, et al. (2007). Prevalence of depression in older people in England and Wales: the MRC CFA Study. *Psychological Medicine*, 37(12): 1787–1795.

Mental Capacity Act 2005, c. 9. Available at: https://www.legislation.gov.uk/ukpga/2005/9/contents [accessed 27th June 2022].

Mental Capacity Act (Northern Ireland) 2016. Available at: https://www.legislation.gov.uk/nia/2016/18/contents/enacted [accessed 17th May 2024].

Mental Health Act 1983, c. 20. Available at: https://www.legislation.gov.uk/ukpga/1983/20/contents [accessed 27th June 2023].

Mental Health (Care and Treatment) (Scotland) Act 2003. Available at: https://www.legislation.gov.uk/asp/2003/13/contents [accessed 17th May 2024].

Mental Health (Northern Ireland) Order 1986. Available at: https://www.legislation.gov.uk/nisi/1986/595/contents [accessed 17th May 2024].

NHS England (2022). Appropriate prescribing of antipsychotic medication in dementia. Available at: https://www.england.nhs.uk/london/wp-content/uploads/sites/8/2022/10/Antipsychotic-Prescribing-Toolkit-for-Dementia.pdf [accessed 22nd April 2024].

O'Brien JT, Thomas A (2015). Vascular dementia. *The Lancet*, 386(10004): 1698–1706.

Pappadà A, et al. (2021). Assistive technologies in dementia care: an updated analysis of the literature. *Frontiers in Psychology*, 12: 644587.

Robertson C (2022). Delirium and dementia. In *Mental Health Care in Paramedic Practice*, Rolfe and Partlow (eds.). Bridgwater: Class Professional Publishing: 137–148.

Rockwood K, et al. (2005). A global clinical measure of fitness and frailty in elderly people. *Canadian Medical Association Journal*, 175(5): 489–495.

Scheltens P, et al. (2021). Alzheimer's disease. *The Lancet*, 397(10284): 1577–1590.

Shepperd S, et al. (2022). Hospital at home admission avoidance with comprehensive geriatric assessment to maintain living at home for people aged 65 years and over: a RCT. *Health and Social Care Delivery Research*, 10(2): 35129936.

Steinert C, et al. (2014). The prospective long-term course of adult depression in general practice and the community. A systematic literature review. *Journal of Affective Disorders*, 152–154: 65–75.

Suen YN, et al. (2019). Late-onset psychosis and very-late-onset-schizophrenia-like-psychosis: an updated systematic review. *International Review of Psychiatry*, 31(5–6): 523–542.

Troya MI, et al. (2019). Self-harm in older adults: systematic review. *The British Journal of Psychiatry*, 214(4): 186–200.

Tsoi KKF, et al. (2015). Cognitive tests to detect dementia: a systematic review and meta-analysis. *JAMA Internal Medicine*, 175(9): 1450–1458.

van der Flier WM, Scheltens P (2005). Epidemiology and risk factors of dementia. *Journal of Neurology, Neurosurgery and Psychiatry*, 76: v2–v7.

Wand APF, et al. (2018). Understanding self-harm in older people: a systematic review of qualitative studies. *Aging and Mental Health*, 22(3): 289–298.

Wolitzky-Taylor KB, et al. (2010). Anxiety disorders in older adults: a comprehensive review. *Depression and Anxiety*, 27(2): 190–211.

Chapter 6

Polypharmacy and Medicines Review

Ruth Harris and Gavin Ronaldson

> **Learning Points**
>
> By the end of this chapter, you will:
>
> - Understand what is meant by 'polypharmacy'
> - Understand the risks of problematic polypharmacy and why older adults living with frailty are more susceptible
> - Understand the key steps involved in medicines review and deprescribing
> - Understand the considerations, challenges and risks to deprescribing medicines.

> **Case Study**
>
> **Background:** You are working in a falls clinic in general practice and see a patient, Brampton (86 years old), who attends with their partner for a structured medicines review as a part of a multidisciplinary falls assessment.
>
> **Presenting Complaint:** On entering the room, you notice that Brampton is unsteady on their feet, requiring support under one elbow by their partner.
>
> **History of Presenting Complaint:** Brampton had a prolonged hospital admission for pneumonia six months ago and has fallen six to seven times since discharge. During their admission, several changes were made to their medication regimen, which was dispensed in a blister pack.
>
> **Past Medical History:** Hypertension, ischaemic heart disease, AFib, type 2 diabetes, congestive heart failure, osteoarthritis of the knees, frailty.
>
> **Allergies:** Tramadol (hallucinations).
>
> **Drug History:** Aspirin (75 mg once daily), apixaban (5 mg twice daily), atorvastatin (80 mg once daily at night), bisoprolol (10 mg once daily), amlodipine (10 mg

CHAPTER 6 Polypharmacy and Medicines Review

once daily), ramipril (2.5 mg once daily), oxybutynin (5 mg twice daily), metformin (1 g twice daily), gliclazide (80 mg twice daily), dapagliflozin (10 mg once daily), co-codamol (30/500 mg four times a day, when required), furosemide (20 mg twice daily), omeprazole (20 mg once daily).

Social History: Lives with partner in a two-bed bungalow, occasional alcohol, no formal POC, partner supports with some ADLs.

Assessment: Brampton appears thin, with loose-fitting clothes. They have a slow walking speed and require support from their partner. They are short of breath walking from the clinic waiting room which resolves quickly on resting and they can speak in full sentences. They are oriented to person, time and place. Brampton is supported with taking medicines by their partner, both of whom have been struggling since the recent hospital admission, as Brampton returned home notably deconditioned, with numerous medication changes that were not clearly explained.

Lying BP: 106/68 mmHg.

Standing BP: 86/60 mmHg.

Heart Rate: 56 bpm.

Temperature: 36.7°C.

Capillary Oxygen Saturations: 94% (room air).

Respiratory Rate: 16 breaths per minute.

Frailty: Rockwood CFS Score 5.

When asked how they have been since hospital discharge, Brampton reports increased drowsiness, dizziness on standing and lacking in energy.

Brampton is pleased to have been invited in for the review, as they both think Brampton is taking too many medicines and they would be keen to stop taking what is no longer necessary.

Initial Impression: Falls, probable orthostatic hypotension, advancing frailty and deconditioning.

Initial Plan: Comprehensive medicines reconciliation. Structured medication review, considering patient's wishes and shared, informed decision making.

Introduction

Throughout the world, medicines remain one of the most important and common interventions in healthcare systems. In this chapter, we will be looking at medicines use in the older adult living with frailty, thinking about polypharmacy, adverse drug reactions (ADRs) and tools to review and rationalise medicines usage to reduce harm.

What is Polypharmacy?

Polypharmacy describes the situation whereby an individual is taking multiple medicines concurrently. Medical texts as far back as the 1800s advise that polypharmacy is something that must be avoided (Royal Pharmaceutical Society, 2022). The Royal Pharmaceutical Society (RPS) recommends that all healthcare professionals have a responsibility to identify polypharmacy and address the issues that it causes (RPS, 2022). Furthermore, it is now a requirement of general practitioners (GPs) to routinely identify and support older adults living with frailty, with a focus on medicines review (NHSE, 2017). This begs the question, how many medicines is too many?

Polypharmacy has been defined as taking anywhere from two to ten medicines at once, with the most used definition being any treatment regimen consisting of five or more medicines (Masnoon et al., 2017). However, with internationally recommended treatment regimens for conditions, such as myocardial infarction (MI) or tuberculosis infection, consisting of at least five different medicines at initiation, this definition becomes less workable (NICE, 2016a; 2020). This also assumes that patients have one condition being treated, whereas, in reality, older adults living with frailty are known to have multiple comorbidities and are likely to be prescribed well over five medicines to manage these.

It can be helpful to frame polypharmacy, in terms of the appropriateness of the medicines prescribed, rather than simply the number (Allan et al., 2019). Appropriate polypharmacy occurs when practitioners combine best available evidence and clinical judgement with the patient's values and preferences, along with an assessment of what is realistic for that individual. Problematic polypharmacy occurs when multiple medicines are prescribed without considering the patients' wishes or ability to take the medicine, where intended benefits are not realised and where risks of ADRs and negative outcomes are high (The King's Fund, 2013).

As clinicians, we need to be alert to the potential of problematic polypharmacy developing from initiation of a new medicine and at any point of the treatment journey. Polypharmacy, be it appropriate or problematic, relies on a combination of three factors. We will discuss each of these in turn:

- Patient
- Medicine
- Disease.

CHAPTER 6 Polypharmacy and Medicines Review

Patient

Life expectancy continues to rise (Knight and Nigam, 2008c), with the complex machine that is the human body running for a lot longer than it would have in years gone by, often without any replacement parts. Even without the burden of disease, organs will age and with this naturally decline in function. Genetic predisposition, lifestyle factors, socioeconomic status and disease, however, play a role in changing the trajectory of this ageing process. Some of these changes in relation to pharmacokinetics are outlined in Figure 6.1 and the following text.

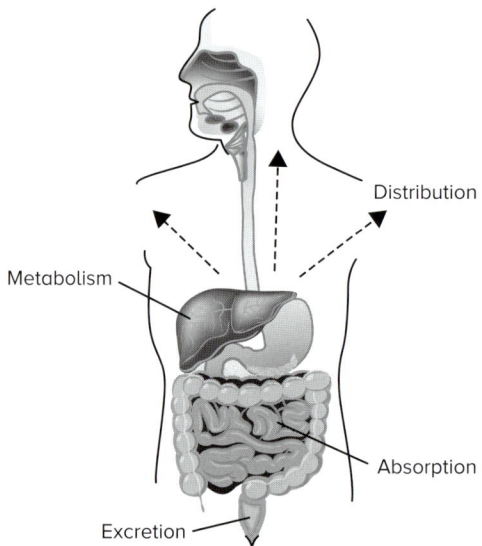

Figure 6.1 The principles of pharmacokinetics.

Absorption

This is the process by which a drug moves from site of administration to systemic circulation. It involves the stomach, small and large intestine, skin and lungs.

Changes in ageing:

- Slowed gastric emptying and reduced peristalsis caused by muscle weakness can delay or prolong onset of action.
- Decreased intestinal surface area.
- Increased gastric pH can impact absorption of drug requiring an acidic environment or may cause dissolution of special tablet coatings (for example enteric coating) earlier than designed (Nigam and Knight, 2008a).
- Skin dehydration and loss of subcutaneous fat layer alter passive diffusion of drugs through the skin (Nigam and Knight, 2008b).
- Loss of alveolar elasticity causes a flattening in structure and reduces surface area for inhaled drugs (Knight and Nigam, 2008a).

Distribution

This is the process by which a drug moves about the body, between systemic circulation to body water, tissues and organs. It involves the heart, vascular system, muscles and lymphatic system.

Changes in ageing:

- Total body water and lean muscle mass decrease, causing a relative increase in body fat and altering the distribution of water-soluble and fat-soluble drugs (Knight et al. 2017).
- Reduced circulating albumin in the blood reduces available protein for drugs that move through the body bound to a protein carrier. This increases the amount of free drug whichs can cause toxicity in usually highly protein bound drugs (Lavan and Gallagher, 2016).
- Decreased cardiac output and thickening and stiffening of blood vessels leads to sluggish blood flow around the body, decreased perfusion of organs and reduced distribution of drugs (Knight and Nigam, 2008c).
- Sluggish lymphatic drainage can cause accumulation of a drug or drugs in body tissues (Lavan and Gallagher, 2016).

Metabolism

This is the process by which a drug is altered by the body; either to become its active form or as a breakdown process before excretion. It involves the liver and the small and large intestine.

Changes in ageing:

- Liver shrinkage caused by hepatocyte (liver cell) death reduces enzyme production. As these enzymes play a critical role in drug metabolism, processing of drugs may be prolonged, or reduced, which means that a person can be exposed to the effects of a drug for much longer than intended. Conversely, where a drug is changed from an inactive form to an active one, a drug may have a delayed onset of action.
- Bacterial flora imbalance and reduced enzyme production can impact drug processing in the small and large intestines (Nigam and Knight, 2008a).

Excretion

This is the process by which the drug is removed from the body. It involves the kidneys, small and large intestine, lungs and skin.

Changes in ageing:

- Reduced kidney size, diminished perfusion and decreasing nephron function cause a gradual age-related decline in renal function. As urinary excretion is the main route of drug elimination, this can be critical to the risk of drug

CHAPTER 6 Polypharmacy and Medicines Review

accumulation and/or toxicity. Natural age-related decline can be exacerbated by disease-related damage in conditions such as cardiovascular disease and type 2 diabetes, both of which are commonly linked to ageing (Lavan and Gallagher, 2016).

- Slowed gastric function and constipation can delay faecal excretion of drugs; the longer a drug stays in the bowel, the greater the risk that some is reabsorbed as circulating levels decline, prolonging the action (Nigam and Knight, 2008a).

- Reduced respiratory effort and alveolar surface area can reduce the efficiency of drugs excreted in respiration (Knight and Nigam, 2008a).

- Impaired thermoregulation and reduced sweat gland function can impact on the efficiency of a drug's excretion via sweat (Knight and Nigam, 2008d).

Prescribing and the Decisions Required

Even when all best evidence is used to prescribe, or deprescribe, a medicine a patient can be at risk of problematic polypharmacy if they do not take a medicine as intended, or be at risk of disease progression or worsening symptoms if they do not take it at all (Allan et al., 2019).

Prescribing should be a collaborative process between patient and clinician; a patient should understand the potential benefits and risks of taking a medicine before making an informed choice and be given the relevant information on how to take the medicine appropriately and safely (NICE, 2021). This is particularly important for medicines that are delivered by devices, such as inhalers, patches or drops, or medicines with specific safety instructions, like alendronic acid (Joint Formulary Committee, 2024).

Sensory or cognitive decline should be considered when making a prescribing decision too (Knight and Nigam, 2008d; Nigam and Knight, 2008e). A patient may understand how to take a medicine appropriately, but may be unable to, due to dexterity issues or an impaired swallow. In these instances, alternative formulations or devices that the patient can use should be considered, seeking advice from pharmacy professionals where necessary.

In the case of cognitive impairment, concordance can be supported with a medical compliance aid as a prompt. The use of an medical compliance aid should be reviewed prior to initiation to ensure the patient and/or their carer can correctly and safely use the device. Medicines will also need to be reviewed to ensure they are compatible with dispensing outside of the manufacturer's original packaging (Community Pharmacy England, 2022).

In special circumstances, where patients lack capacity to make decisions about whether or not to take their medicines, a best interests decision can be made by the MDT and a patient's representative to give medicines covertly (that is, administered via a patient's food or drink). However, this practice should be avoided unless necessary and in line with relevant policies and guidelines (Specialist Pharmacy Service, 2024). Advice from pharmacy professionals should be sought when manipulating any medicines formulations for covert administration.

Medicine

> 'I take metformin for the diabetes, caused by the bendroflumethiazide I take for high blood pressure, which I got from the citalopram I take for anxiety, that I got from methylphenidate I take for chronic fatigue, which I got from the atorvastatin I take because I have high cholesterol, because it's difficult to find time for diet and exercise!'

Adverse Drug Reactions

Occasionally, an unwanted or harmful reaction can occur. This is an adverse drug reaction (ADR) (Medicines and Healthcare products Regulatory Agency (MHRA), 2022). Table 6.1 outlines the five types of reactions.

An ADR can occur because of a single medicine or a combination of two or more co-administered and can be complicated by patient or disease-specific factors.

ADRs can be categorised into five types:

Table 6.1 Common types of reactions.

Reaction Type	Description
Type A (augmented) reactions:	An exaggerated, or augmented, response to the known or expected effects of medicine(s) taken at the usual dose is a Type A ADR. The effects can either be the intended therapeutic outcome (such as bleeding with anticoagulants, like warfarin or apixaban, or gliclazide causing hypoglycaemia), or a known or common side effect (such as a dry cough with ramipril).
	In the context of older individuals living with frailty, type A ADRs may occur where two or more medicines with the same therapeutic use may have an additive effect (such as amlodipine, ramipril and indapamide being concurrently prescribed for hypertension, but instead causing hypotension).
	Type A ADRs are usually dose dependent, which means the unwanted effects tend to reduce on dose reduction or stop once the medicine(s) are ceased.

CHAPTER 6 Polypharmacy and Medicines Review

Table 6.1 Common types of reactions (*Continued*).

Reaction Type	Description
Type B (bizarre) reactions:	Type B ADRs are unpredictable, unexpected and thankfully, rare. They are not necessarily related to the pharmacological action of the medicine and can include anaphylaxis, skin rashes or facial swelling upon starting a new medicine.
Type C (continuing) reactions:	Type C ADRs are persistent, enduring effects caused by medicines that are not reversible such as osteonecrosis of the jaw with long-term bisphosphonates, like alendronate. In older individuals living with frailty that may have taken some medicines for a significant amount of time, it is important to be alert to the risk of Type C ADRs. Risk of Type C ADRs can be reduced with clear documentation of the starting date (including year) of a medicine in an individual's clinical notes and routine (at least annual) medicines review.
Type D (delayed) reactions:	Type D ADRs are those that do not necessarily occur while an individual is taking a medicine. Instead, these reactions may manifest days, weeks or months after the treatment has ended. Type D ADRs are commonly associated with chemotherapy treatments, where they may include abnormalities in blood counts that appear days or weeks after a chemotherapy dose, or the development of a new cancer years after successful treatment of a different cancer.
Type E (end-of-use) reactions:	Type E ADRs are usually withdrawal-related reactions. Medicines which are most likely to cause these ADRs are those that either increase or decrease the amount of enzymes or neurotransmitters in the body, such as antidepressants (like sertraline, amitriptyline) or benzodiazepines (diazepam or lorazepam). The Type E ADR occurs due to the body trying to readjust to life without the medicine. The risk of Type E ADRs is reduced by slow withdrawal, or tapering of dosages, rather than stopping these medicines suddenly.

It stands to reason that the more medicines a person takes, the more likely they are to experience an ADR (Allan et al., 2019): a person taking two medicines has a 13% risk of experiencing an ADR, increasing to an 82% risk when taking seven or more medicines concurrently (Lavan and Gallagher, 2016; Zazzara et al., 2021). ADRs are known to significantly impact morbidity and mortality and, with nearly two million older adults in the UK taking at least seven medicines a day, there is a huge proportion of people at significant risk of harm or death because of the medicines they are prescribed (Age UK, 2019).

Occasionally, an ADR is mistaken for the symptom of a pre-existing condition or a new health concern, leading to prescribing of another medicine to reverse or remove this symptom. This is called a prescribing cascade (Rochon and Gurwitz, 1997) (Figure 6.2).

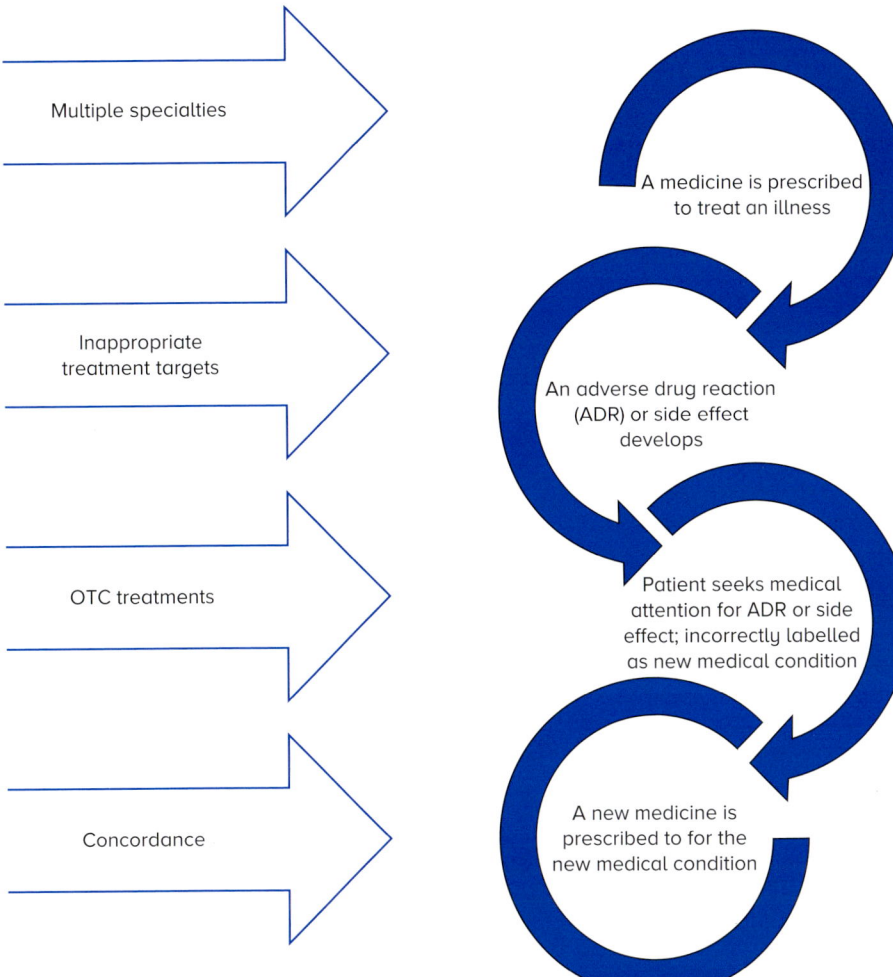

Figure 6.2 The prescribing cascade.
Source: Adapted from Rochon and Gurwitz, 1997.

In older adults living with frailty, prescribing cascades can be compounded by several other factors including:

- Multiple specialties treating individual conditions: do not always consider the impact of other treatments or organ systems
- Unrealistic targets: adding more medicines in to achieve treatment targets that may not be suitable for the patient
- Concordance: assuming patients take medication as prescribed when in fact they do not, meaning extra medicines are added as it appears treatment targets (and potentially unrealistic targets) are not being achieved
- Over-the-counter (OTC) and patient choice; patients doing things clinicians may not be aware of.

CHAPTER 6   Polypharmacy and Medicines Review

ADRs – Why Worry About Them?

ADRs can negatively impact on quality of life and adversely affect concordance to medicines, which may compromise the patient-prescriber relationship (The King's Fund, 2013). Data from the early 2000s suggested that ADRs were responsible for approximately 6.5% of hospital admissions in the UK (Allan et al., 2019; Pirmohamed and Park, 2003) with over 70% of these being avoidable. More recent data (Osanlou et al., 2022) demonstrated an increase in this figure, with ADRs now accounting for around 16% of hospital admissions with around 40% potentially being avoidable. An older person living with even a mild degree of frailty is twice as likely to develop an ADR during an admission (Zazzara et al., 2021) and are almost twice as likely to develop an ADR than younger adults (Lavan and Gallagher, 2016).

The vast majority (80%) of ADRs are Type A ADRs, with Types B–E making up the other 20%. This means that most ADRs can not only be predicted, but can also be reduced or avoided entirely. The key to this risk reduction or avoidance is knowledge. Any actual or suspected ADR should be reported using the MHRA Yellow Card Scheme. Reports can be submitted online via the Yellow Card website, through a mobile app, by phone or by completing a paper form.

Disease

Diseases in older people present more subtly and atypically than their younger, non-frail counterparts (Gupta and Bhomwick, 2010). They can report what the British Geriatrics Society (BGS) categorises as non-specific complaints; that is, symptoms caused by the interaction between a person's underlying comorbidities and associated polypharmacy (BGS, 2021).

The concern is that where these non-specific complaints draw no definitive diagnosis, older people living with frailty can undergo multiple tests and investigations that may arguably not change the outcome of their circumstances, yet increase the risk of harm, injury and undue stress (Gupta and Bhomwick, 2010).

Often, treatment specific guidelines call for escalating therapies as a chronic condition progresses, however, very old people living with frailty may experience severe or end-stage disease, at which point some medicines started at earlier stages may now be obsolete (in other words, disease burden exceeds any benefit that can be derived from the medicines prescribed for it) or requiring such high doses of a medicine that side effects or ADRs may outweigh any benefit from the intended action of the medicine (Lavan et al., 2017; Scottish Government Polypharmacy Model of Care Group, 2018).

It is important to take stock of a patient's medicines regime at each LTC review, as well as symptom management and signs of disease progression.

Medicine Reviews and Deprescribing

When Should a Medicine Review Take Place?

Older adults living with frailty should have an annual structured medication review with a suitably skilled practitioner. In addition to this regular review, any acute clinical change in a patient resulting in an encounter with a healthcare professional should prompt an opportunistic review of a patient's medications to rule out their usage as a potential cause for harm.

Should a first responder feel a medicines review is required, but is unable to undertake this themselves, they should make a specific onward recommendation to the receiving clinical team to ensure this is undertaken as part of a referral pathway or handover. Available resources and services should be discussed with your local primary and secondary care providers.

Medicines Reconciliation and History Taking

To review a patient's treatment, it is vital that an up-to-date list of all the medicines a person is taking is collated. This process, commonly known as medicines reconciliation (NICE, 2015), should cover all details of a patients' medicines history including:

- Those prescribed by healthcare professionals
- Any long-term medicines recently stopped
- Any short/acute courses of medicines
- OTC products
- Herbal and dietary supplements including complementary medicine and illicit/recreational substances
- Any known allergies or intolerances to medicines.

The dosage, dosing frequency and route of administration should also be documented as well as details of when the medicine was started and the indication for the medicine being prescribed. Remember to ask about medicines that are often forgotten about such as inhalers, eye drops and topical preparations. When considering the indication for each medicine, information relating to when and how the medical condition was diagnosed should be documented as this may influence future decisions around continuing or stopping the medicine in question.

When undertaking medicines reconciliation, several sources of information are available and it is recommended that more than one source is used (NICE, 2015). In the context of older adults living with frailty, given the increased prevalence of polypharmacy and complexity of medicine regimens, it is vital that either the patient, or somebody involved in the care and/or administration of a patients' medicines, is consulted. With an estimated 30–50% of medicines not being taken as prescribed (NICE, 2016b), relying solely on healthcare records may result in inaccurate and incomplete information.

Sources of information for collating a medicine history:

- Patient or next of kin
- Carer involved in administration of medicines
- Patient's own medicines (if conveying a patient from their place of residence to hospital ensure these are transferred with the patient)

CHAPTER 6 Polypharmacy and Medicines Review

- GP records and Summary Care Record (SCR)
- Hospital discharge letters
- District nursing notes
- Medicines Administration Record (MAR).

Principles of Undertaking a Medicines Review and Deprescribing

While several tools for undertaking a medicine review exist, for the purposes of this chapter we will focus primarily on the NHS Scotland (2018) '7 Steps to Appropriate Polypharmacy' model.

Step 1 – What Matters to the Patient

Shared decision making should underpin all decisions relating to the prescribing and deprescribing of medicines. Evidence has shown that when patients are involved in decisions about their treatment, they are more likely to adhere to decisions made and have positive healthcare outcomes.

An understanding of the patient's personal perspective on managing their medicines is a key stage in the process. A particular focus should be on how managing medicines fits into their daily routine (Barnett et al., 2016). It should also be noted that a patient's desired treatment outcomes may differ from that of the clinician; for example, patients may focus on functional benefits such as being able to see friends or family rather than specific treatment targets or levels of risk reduction. Shared decision making allows both parties to communicate their expectations and reach a mutually agreed decision.

When engaging patients in discussions about their treatment, it is essential to outline the potential benefits and risks of a given intervention. This can be quantified by using data on numbers needed to treat (NNT) and numbers needed to harm (NNH). No medicine is 100% effective nor is any medicine completely free from risk of harm, and several datasets exist to display this information. Patient decision aids for specific interventions can be used to involve patients in decisions about their medicines.

Finally, licensing constraints and progressions of disease state should also be considered when reviewing medicines. Some medicines may have a limited evidence base or not be recommended once a clinical condition has progressed beyond a certain point. Similarly, the potential risks and benefits when using a medicine to prevent disease should be reviewed, particularly when the evidence informing clinical practice may be based on time specific mortality data that extends beyond the expected lifespan of the patient.

A common example of this is statins being prescribed for the secondary prevention of cardiovascular disease, whose evidence is based on five and ten-year mortality data (NICE, 2023). That said, emerging evidence (Giral et al., 2019) has shown that statins may continue to be beneficial in older patients, which highlights the importance of clinicians remaining up to date with guidance and engaging patients in meaningful conversations about their medicines to ensure they can make an informed decision.

Steps 2 and 3 – Identify Essential and Unnecessary Medicines

When determining the necessity of a given medicine, in addition to the patient's views, there are two important factors to consider:

1. Does the medicine replace a normal physiological requirement (for example levothyroxine in hypothyroidism)?
2. Does the medicine prevent rapid symptomatic decline of a medical condition (for example medicines used in the management of Parkinson's disease)?

If the answer to either of these questions is yes, then specialist advice should be sought before any alteration to, or cessation of, these medicines. Following on from the above, with each medicine, the following considerations should be made:

- Is there still a valid indication for the prescribed medicine and is treatment still being prescribed in line with current, evidence-based practice?
- Has the disease progressed since the initial prescribing of the medicine and is treatment still considered appropriate?
- Is the medicine being used to manage current symptoms, prolong life expectancy or as secondary prevention of an acute event?
- Are medicines being continued to achieve a mortality reduction benefit that may exceed a patient's life expectancy?
- Are the formulation, dose and dosing frequency still appropriate for the patient?

When reviewing the necessity of individual medicines, several other tools and resources are available to aid clinicians and their patients in making informed decisions concerning their treatment (Table 6.2).

Table 6.2 Tools to aid medication review.

Resource	Comments
Beers criteria (American Geriatrics Society, 2019)	Provides information on stopping/reducing medicines in older people. American resource: UK practice may differ.
STOPP/START (Rochon et al., 2023)	Part of the CGA toolkit; this supports medicines optimisation, focusing on identifying appropriate medicines to prescribe/deprescribe in older people.
STOPPFrail (Lavan et al., 2017)	A tool focusing on review of medicines in older people living with frailty. Guidance on considering long-term benefits of medicines against a patient's prognosis.
MedStopper (MedStopper, 2023)	Where there are a number of medicines that are to be stopped, this automated calculator provides advice on prioritising which medicines to review first.

Step 4 – Review Therapeutic Objectives

As clinicians we must also outline the intended therapeutic goals for prescribing medicines. Depending on the type of medicine and intended indication, the therapeutic objectives may vary and could include, but are not limited to:

- Symptom control, for example, proton pump inhibitors in gastro-oesophageal reflux disease
- Replacement of a normal physiological function, for example, insulin in the management of type 1 diabetes
- Prevention in disease progression or complications from medical condition, for example, antiretroviral use in the management of HIV
- Primary or secondary prevention of disease, for example, bisphosphonates for the prevention of fragility fractures
- Distinct treatment target, for example, HbA1c targets in the management of type 2 diabetes
- Treatment of active disease pathology, for example, antibiotics for urinary tract infection.

Some medicines may serve to meet more than one therapeutic objective.

When reviewing the therapeutic objectives in the context of an older adult living with frailty, it is imperative that the initial aims of treatment are still relevant and valid. Consider, for example, if symptoms are being adequately controlled by medicines and, if not, is their continuation justifiable. Likewise, consider if the original cause for a given symptom is still present and therefore if the medicine is still needed, such as exercise-induced angina in a patient who now has limited mobility and the need to continue isosorbide mononitrate, which may increase the risk of falls.

Where distinct, measurable outcomes are available, such as blood pressure readings, clinicians should review what parameters are deemed acceptable in the context of a patient living with frailty. In the management of blood glucose control for patients with diabetes, the Association of British Clinical Diabetologists (2019) recommend higher target HbA1c values to reduce the risk of complications from hypoglycaemia. Similarly, research has shown that raising blood pressure targets for frail patients has a positive impact on mortality, suggesting that in patients over 75 years of age, reducing systolic blood pressure below 130 mmHg may not be suitable due to increased risk of adverse events (Masoli et al., 2020).

Step 5 – Identify Potential/Actual ADRs

Medicines use may contribute to any one of the known frailty syndromes and should be considered as a potential cause of any newly reported symptoms to avoid prescribing cascades. A mixture of open and closed questions, as well as probing questions, should be used when discussing adverse effects to identify their presence and potential cause.

Of particular concern to the population living with frailty is the risk of falls, a risk which can often be exacerbated by the use of medicine (Ziere et al., 2006). The Royal College of Physicians (RCP) FallSafe tool (RCP, 2015; The Health Foundation, 2015) highlights the three main mechanisms by which medicines can contribute to falls and details key medicines which may contribute, grading them using a traffic light system. It allows users to quickly identify medicines that may increase the risk of falls, although it does not provide guidance on how or when to stop these medicines nor does it consider the other considerations outlined in this chapter.

Another area of increasing concern is the cumulative impact of medications with anticholinergic effects, with recent studies linking their use to cognitive decline (Richardson et al., 2018). Other known effects of anticholinergic drugs include dry eyes and visual disturbances, dry mouth, constipation and urinary retention, postural hypotension and heart rhythm disturbances (Joint National Formulary, 2024). While some medicines may be prescribed specifically for their anticholinergic properties, such as in the management of overactive bladder, others may have incidental anticholinergic activity which is distinct from their intended therapeutic use. Consequently, it is not just an individual medicine's activity that must be considered, but rather the cumulative effect of all the medicines a person takes; a concept known as the anticholinergic burden. Several online tools are available to assess an individual's anticholinergic burden, as well as strategies to reduce this score and thus potential harm (Table 6.3).

Table 6.3 Anticholinergic burden (ACB) calculators.

Resource	Comments
ACB Calculator (King and Rabino, 2023)	Typing in names of medicines will create an aggregate ACB score, while also giving information about the ACB score of each individual medicine. It also provides some supportive quantitative evidence for the relevance of ACB scoring.
Medichec (South London and Maudsley NHS Foundation Trust, 2024)	Typing in names of medicines will create an aggregate ACB score, while also giving information about the ACB score of each individual medicine. Also provides relative potency of dizziness/drowsiness as side effects of each medicine.

Step 6 – Cost Effectiveness

When considering the cost effectiveness of a given treatment, your local medicines management services or prescribing committees can advise on the most appropriate prescribing decisions. A key point to remember is that the most ineffective use of resources is a medicine that the patient is unable or unwilling to take. Furthermore, in some circumstances, for example in the management of epilepsy, it is vital that patients are not switched between different brands or formulations of medicine without prior specialist review (MHRA, 2017).

CHAPTER 6 Polypharmacy and Medicines Review

Step 7 – Agree and Share Plan

Once potentially inappropriate polypharmacy has been identified, the final steps are planning how this will be addressed and sharing this plan with all relevant parties involved in managing the patient's medicines.

When looking to stop medicines, it is imperative that a stepwise approach is taken, reducing, or stopping, one medicine at a time and assessing the impact before deprescribing another. If two or more medicines are adjusted concurrently and adverse effects occur, it becomes difficult to ascertain which intervention may have led to the unwanted outcome. Similarly, it is vital to know – before making any adjustment – which medicines can be stopped abruptly and which may require a slower tapering of dose prior to cessation, seeking specialist advice where necessary.

Other barriers to deprescribing medicines relate to patients' perceptions of how their medicines benefit them and the language used when discussing stopping them (Doherty et al., 2020). Choice of language is crucial when communicating options, considering use of phrases such as 'trial without' rather than 'stopping'. Many of these issues can be overcome by giving appropriate information on expected duration of treatment when starting medicines, particularly avoiding terms such as 'lifelong'.

Providing safety-netting advice and mechanisms to deal with adverse effects from withdrawing a medicine are also likely to help in successfully rationalising inappropriate polypharmacy. In addition, for some medicines, a treatment break or 'drug holiday' may also be beneficial, a practice commonly seen where bisphosphonates are used in the management of osteoporosis for the prevention of fragility fractures (National Osteoporosis Guideline Group, 2021).

The final step to successfully deprescribing medicines is communication of the plan to the patient and those involved with their care as failure to do so may result in changes not being sustained or medicine errors occurring. A particularly problematic area where this occurs is at the transfer of patients across boundaries of care, with an estimated 30–70% risk of unintentional changes to medication occurring at this point in a patient's journey (RPS, 2012). When communicating changes to medications, assess whether any of the following need to be contacted (ensuring appropriate data-sharing agreements are in place and in accordance with the General Data Protection Regulation (GDPR)):

- Patient and next of kin
- Primary care provider (GP, practice nurse, practice pharmacist)
- Community pharmacist
- District nursing teams
- Social care providers, especially if involved in administration of medicines
- Specialist clinical teams involved in the patient's care
- Voluntary sector organisations.

It must also be noted that the medication review process is not a linear process and the patient should be reviewed regularly, particularly if changes to medicines are made or if the clinical condition of the patient changes over time.

Further Considerations

Patients should be deemed to have capacity unless proven otherwise and capacity should be reassessed at each encounter before making any prescribing decisions. As previously discussed, certain medicines may contribute to an acute delirium or a cognitive decline and stopping or withdrawing these may affect future capacity assessments. Where lack of capacity has been established, an MDT approach should be taken to discuss what is in the best interests of a patient, including a review of any advance care plans and the input of any lasting power of attorney(s) for health and well-being, the patient's next of kin or an independent mental capacity advocate.

Before making any decision to deprescribe a medicine, the legal implications of doing so should also be borne in mind. Any decision to deprescribe a medicine should be treated with the same level of diligence as a decision to prescribe a medicine and should only be done by a clinician with the appropriate skills and qualifications to do so.

Finally, it is important to remember that there may be circumstances where older adults living with frailty may benefit from the addition of new treatments to their current regimen. As previously discussed, evidence-based medicine and shared decision making is imperative when making decisions to start a new medicine in an older adult living with frailty.

Conclusion

This chapter highlighted some of the risks associated with inappropriate polypharmacy and the physiological changes that occur with ageing that can predispose patients to the harmful effects of medicines. It also outlined some of the key elements to consider when undertaking a medicines review.

To successfully rationalise a patient's medicines and reduce the risk of harm, communication is key. Firstly, by engaging in open conversations with patients and their caregivers about the use of medications and desired treatment outcomes, shared decisions can be made regarding the continued use of these medicines. Secondly, by agreeing a plan and sharing this information amongst the wider team involved in a patient's care, we can ensure that any changes to treatment are continued and appropriate safety netting is in place should any adverse events occur.

Given the complexities associated with medicines use in the frail population, it is vital that services designed to support this cohort of patients have pharmacy teams included within the MDT.

CHAPTER 6 Polypharmacy and Medicines Review

> **What Are Your Thoughts on Brampton's Medicines List?**
>
> 1. Can you detect any signs of a prescribing cascade in Brampton's medicines list?
> 2. Considering the 7-steps process, look back at Brampton, their medical history and medicines list; are there opportunities to rationalise their medicines to reduce the risk of harm?
> 3. Looking at Brampton's medicines list, is there potential for Type A ADRs?

Further Resources

Polypharmacy and Medicines Review

- Allan F, Guthrie B and Kelman A (2019). Polypharmacy: A framework for theory and practice. *The Pharmaceutical Journal.* Available at: https://pharmaceutical-journal.com/article/ld/polypharmacy-a-framework-for-theory-and-practice

- Duerden M, Avery T and Payne R (2013). *Polypharmacy and Medicines Optimisation: Making it safe and sound.* The King's Fund. Available at: https://www.kingsfund.org.uk/publications/polypharmacy-and-medicinesoptimisation

- National Institute for Health and Care Excellence (NICE) (2015). *Medicines optimisation: The safe and effective use of medicines to enable the best possible outcomes.* Available at: https://www.nice.org.uk/guidance/ng5/resources/medicines-optimisation-the-safe-and-effective-use-of-medicines-to-enable-the-best-possible-outcomespdf-51041805253

- Scottish Government Polypharmacy Model of Care Group (2018). *Polypharmacy Guidance, Realistic Prescribing (3rd edition).* Scottish Government. Available at: https://www.therapeutics.scot.nhs.uk/wp-content/uploads/2018/04/Polypharmacy-Guidance-2018.pdf

Non-Medical Prescribing

- Royal Pharmaceutical Society (2021). *A Competency Framework for All Prescribers*: https://www.rpharms.com/resources/frameworks/prescribing-competency-framework/competency-framework

- Blaber et al. (2018). *Independent prescribing for paramedics.* Bridgwater: Class Professional Publishing.

- Rutt-Howard and Nuttall (2011). *The textbook of non-medical prescribing.* London: Wiley Blackwell.

Condition-Specific Resources

- National Osteoporosis Guideline Group (2021). *Clinical Guideline for the Prevention and Treatment of Osteoporosis*: https://www.nogg.org.uk/full-guideline

- Strain et Al. (2021). Diabetes and Frailty: An Expert Consensus Statement on the Management of Older Adults with Type 2 Diabetes. *Diabetes Therapy*, 12: 1227–1247.

- National Institute for Health and Care Excellence (NICE) (2022). Medicines Associated with Dependence or Withdrawal Symptoms: Safe Prescribing and Withdrawal Management for Adults: https://www.nice.org.uk/guidance/ng215/resources/medicines-associated-with-dependence-or-withdrawal-symptoms-safe-prescribing-and-withdrawal-management-for-adults-pdf-66143776880581

- Mallery et al. (2014). Promoting higher blood pressure targets for frail older adults: a consensus guideline from Canada. *Cleveland Clinical Journal of Medicine*, 81(7): 427–437.

- ACB Calculator: https://www.acbcalc.com/

References

Age UK (2019). Age UK calls for a more considered approach to prescribing medicines for our older people. Available at: https://www.ageuk.org.uk/portsmouth/about-us/news/articles/2019/age-uk-calls-for-a-more-considered-approach-to-prescribing-medicines-for-our-older-population [accessed 4th June 2024].

Allan F, Guthrie B, Kelman A (2019). Polypharmacy: a framework for theory and practice. *The Pharmaceutical Journal*. Available at: https://pharmaceutical-journal.com/article/ld/polypharmacy-a-framework-for-theory-and-practice [accessed 6th August 2024].

American Geriatrics Society (2019). Updated AGS Beers criteria® for potentially inappropriate medication use in older adults. *Journal of the American Geriatrics Society*, 67(4): 20190129.

Association of British Clinical Diabetologists (2019). Position statement: Managing frailty and associated comorbidities in older adults with diabetes. Available at: https://abcd.care/sites/default/files/site_uploads/Resources/Position-Papers/ABCD-Position-Paper-Frailty.pdf [accessed 4th June 2024].

Barnett NL, Oboh L, Smith K (2016). Patient-centred management of polypharmacy: a process for practice. *European Journal of Hospital Pharmacy*, 23(2): 113–117.

British Geriatrics Society (2021). *Silver book II: Geriatric syndromes*. Available at: https://www.bgs.org.uk/resources/silver-book-ii-geriatric-syndromes [accessed 4th June 2024].

Community Pharmacy England (2022). Medicines Compliance Assessment Tool. Available at: https://cpe.org.uk/wp-content/uploads/2015/01/19748-Medicines-Compliance-Assessment-Tool.pdf [accessed 11th June 2024].

Doherty AJ, et al. (2020). Barriers and facilitators to deprescribing in primary care: a systematic review. *British Journal of General Practice Open*, 4(3): bjgpopen20X101096.

Giral P, et al. (2019). Cardiovascular effect of discontinuing statins for primary prevention at the age of 75 years: a nationwide population-based cohort study in France. *European Heart Journal*, 40(43): 3516–3525.

Gupta P, Bhomwick B (2010). Ulysses syndrome: unnecessary investigation in older people. *Geriatric Medicine Journal*, 40. Available at: https://pavilionhealthtoday.com/gm/ulysses-syndrome-unnecessary-investigation-in-older-people/ [accessed 6th April 2024].

CHAPTER 6   Polypharmacy and Medicines Review

Joint Formulary Committee (2024). British National Formulary (online). London: BMJ and Pharmaceutical Press. Available at: http://www.medicinescomplete.com [accessed 13th June 2024].

Joint National Formulary (2024). Oxybutynin hydrochloride: British National Formulary. Available at: https://bnf.nice.org.uk/drugs/oxybutynin-hydrochloride/ [accessed 14th June 2024].

King R, Rabino S (2023). ACB calculator. Available at: https://www.acbcalc.com/ [accessed 4th June 2024].

Knight J, Nigam Y (2008a). Exploring the anatomy and physiology of ageing. Part 2 – the respiratory system. *Nursing Times*, 104(32): 24–25.

Knight J, Nigam Y (2008b). Exploring the anatomy and physiology of ageing. Part 10 – muscles and bone. *Nursing Times*, 104(48): 22–23.

Knight J, Nigam Y (2008c). Exploring the anatomy and physiology of ageing. Part 1 – the cardiovascular system. *Nursing Times*, 104(31): 26–27.

Knight J, Nigam Y (2008d). Exploring the anatomy and physiology of ageing. Part 7 – the endocrine system. *Nursing Times*, 104(45): 24–25.

Knight J, Nigam Y (2008e). Exploring the anatomy and physiology of ageing. Part 5 – the nervous system. *Nursing Times*, 104(35): 18–19.

Knight J et al. (2017). Anatomy and physiology of ageing 10: the musculoskeletal system. *Nursing Time*, 113(11): 60–63.

Lavan AH, Gallagher P (2016). Predicting risk of adverse drug reactions in older adults. *Therapeutic Advances in Drug Safety*, 7(1): 11–22.

Lavan AH, et al. (2017). STOPPFrail (Screening Tool of Older Persons Prescriptions in Frail adults with limited life expectancy): consensus validation. *Age and Ageing*, 46(4): 600–607.

Masnoon N, et al. (2017). What is polypharmacy? A systematic review of definitions. *BMC Geriatrics*, 17(1): 20171010.

Masoli JAH, et al. (2020). Blood pressure in frail older adults: associations with cardiovascular outcomes and all-cause mortality. *Age and Ageing*, 49(5): 807–813.

Medicines and Healthcare Products Regulatory Agency (MHRA) (2017). Antiepileptic drugs: updated advice on switching between different manufacturers' products. Available at: https://www.gov.uk/drug-safety-update/antiepileptic-drugs-updated-advice-on-switching-between-different-manufacturers-products [accessed 6th August 2024].

Medicines and Healthcare Products Regulatory Agency (MHRA) (2022). Guidance on adverse drug reactions. Available at: https://assets.publishing.service.gov.uk/media/5feefb4c8fa8f53b7a0fbe36/Guidance_on_adverse_drug_reactions.pdf [accessed 6th August 2024].

MedStopper (2023). Medstopper beta. Available at: https://medstopper.com/ [accessed 6th August 2024].

NHS Scotland (2018). The 7-Steps medication review. Available at: https://rightdecisions.scot.nhs.uk/polypharmacy-guidance/principles/the-7-steps-medication-review/ [accessed 14th October 2024].

National Institute for Health and Care Excellence (NICE) (2015). Medicines optimisation: the safe and effective use of medicines to enable the best possible outcomes (NICE guideline NG5). Available at: https://www.nice.org.uk/guidance/ng5 [accessed 6th August 2024].

National Institute for Health and Care Excellence (NICE) (2016a). Tuberculosis (NICE guideline NG33). Available at: https://www.nice.org.uk/guidance/ng33 [accessed 6th August 2024].

National Institute for Health and Care Excellence (NICE) (2016b). Medicines optimisation (Quality standard QS120). Available at: https://www.nice.org.uk/guidance/qs120 [accessed 6th August 2024].

References

National Institute for Health and Care Excellence (NICE) (2020). Acute coronary syndromes (NICE guideline NG185). Available at: https://www.nice.org.uk/guidance/ng185 [accessed 6th August 2024].

National Institute for Health and Care Excellence (NICE) (2021). Shared decision making (NICE guideline NG197). Available at: https://www.nice.org.uk/guidance/ng197 [accessed 6th August 2024].

National Institute for Health and Care Excellence (NICE) (2023). Cardiovascular disease: risk assessment and reduction, including lipid modification. (NICE guideline NG238). Available at: https://www.nice.org.uk/guidance/ng238 [accessed 6th August 2024].

National Osteoporosis Guideline Group (NOGG) (2021). NOGG 2021: Clinical Guideline for the Prevention and Treatment of Osteoporosis. Available at: https://www.nogg.org.uk/full-guideline [accessed 6th August 2024].

NHSE (2017). Involving people in their own health and care: statutory guidance for clinical commissioning groups and NHS England. Available at: https://www.england.nhs.uk/publication/involving-people-in-their-own-health-and-care-statutory-guidance-for-clinical-commissioning-groups-and-nhs-england/ [accessed 6th August 2024].

Nigam Y, Knight J (2008a). Exploring the anatomy and physiology of ageing. Part 3 – the digestive system. *Nursing Times*, 104(33): 22–23.

Nigam Y, Knight J (2008b). Exploring the anatomy and physiology of ageing. Part 11 – the skin. *Nursing Times*, 104(49): 24–25.

Nigam Y, Knight J (2008c). Exploring the anatomy and physiology of ageing. Part 6 – the eye and ear. *Nursing Times*, 104(36): 22–23.

Osanlou R, et al. (2022). Adverse drug reactions, multimorbidity and polypharmacy: a prospective analysis of 1 month of medical admissions. *British Medical Journal Open*, 12(7): e055551.

Pirmohamed M, Park BK (2003). Adverse drug reactions: back to the future. *British Journal of Clinical Pharmacology*, 55(5): 486–492.

Richardson K, et al. (2018). Anticholinergic drugs and risk of dementia: case-control study. *British Medical Journal*, 361: 20180425.

Rochon PA, et al. (2023). STOPP/START version 3: even better with age. *European Geriatric Medicine*, 14(4): 635–637.

Rochon PA, Gurwitz JH (1997). Optimising drug treatment for elderly people: the prescribing cascade. *British Medical Journal*, 315(7115): 1096–1099.

Royal College of Physicians (RCP) (2015). Medicines and falls in hospital, guidance sheet. Available at: https://www.rcplondon.ac.uk/file/933/download [accessed 6th August 2024].

Royal Pharmaceutical Society (RPS) (2012). Keeping patients safe when they transfer between care providers – getting the medicines right. Available at: https://www.rpharms.com/Portals/0/RPS%20document%20library/Open%20access/Publications/Keeping%20patients%20safe%20transfer%20of%20care%20report.pdf [accessed 6th August 2024].

Royal Pharmaceutical Society (RPS) (2022). Polypharmacy: getting our medicines right. Available at: https://www.rpharms.com/recognition/setting-professional-standards/polypharmacy [accessed 6th August 2024].

Scottish Government Polypharmacy Model of Care Group (2018). *Polypharmacy Guidance, Realistic Prescribing* (3rd edition). Scotland: Scottish Government.

South London and Maudsley NHS Foundation Trust (2024). Medichec Tool. Available at: https://medichec.com/ [accessed 6th August 2024].

Specialist Pharmacy Service (2024). Covert administration of medicines: legal issues. Available at: https://www.sps.nhs.uk/articles/covert-administration-of-medicines-legal-issues/ [accessed 6th August 2024].

CHAPTER 6 Polypharmacy and Medicines Review

The Health Foundation (2015). The FallSafe Project. The Health Foundation. Available at: https://www.health.org.uk/improvement-projects/the-fallsafe-project [accessed 6th August 2024].

The King's Fund (2013). Polypharmacy and medicines optimisation: making it safe and sound. Available at: https://assets.kingsfund.org.uk/f/256914/x/0ffd18f8d6/polypharmacy_medicines_optismisation_2013.pdf [accessed 6th August 2024].

Zazzara MB, et al. (2021). Adverse drug reactions in older adults: a narrative review of the literature. *European Geriatric Medicine*, 12(3): 20210318.

Ziere G, et al. (2006). Polypharmacy and falls in the middle age and elderly population. *British Journal of Clinical Pharmacology*, 61(2): 218–223.

Chapter 7

Activities of Daily Living

Sophie Wallington and Beverley Clare

Learning Points

By the end of this chapter, you will:

- Understand the relationship between acute illness and physical function
- Be able to understand the functional assessment of the older person in the community
- Understand the relationship between a person and their lived environment.

Case Study

Background: You are an urgent care paramedic called to an 89-year-old woman, Hazel, coded as a generally unwell adult. Hazel's home care worker has escalated directly to 999 following a planned home care visit at 10:00 to assist with showering.

Presenting Complaint: Hazel is 'stuck in her chair', unable to independently rise or mobilise. She feels weak and unable to stand due to reduced strength. She is alert and orientated to time, place and person, is following instructions and answering questions clearly and appropriately and does not appear confused.

History of Presenting Complaint: Hazel reports feeling 'off' for the previous few days with slight nausea, reduced fluids and appetite. She has been mobile less around the home, but up until today she has been able to get out of her chair. Last night Hazel fell asleep in her chair and felt too exhausted to go up to bed when she woke. She was able to get up in the night to use the toilet to empty her bladder.

Past Medical History: Hypertension, chronic venous insufficiency with previous leg ulcers, paroxysmal AFib, chronic low back pain (osteoarthritis of the lumbar spine), iron-deficiency anaemia.

CHAPTER 7 Activities of Daily Living

Allergies: No known drug allergies.

Drug History: Ramipril (5 mg once daily), apixaban (5 mg twice daily), lansoprazole (30 mg once daily), bendroflumethiazide (2.5 mg once daily), ferrous fumarate (210 mg twice daily), paracetamol (1 g four times daily), gabapentin (300 mg three times daily), oxycontin (5 mg modified release tablet twice daily), Movicol® (one or two as required).

No history of illicit drug use or OTC supplements or medication.

Social History: Hazel lives alone (her husband died 12 years ago). She has two daughters and one son who visit a few times a month. She rarely leaves the house unless she has medical appointments to attend. She spends her time reading, watching television or listening to the radio. Hazel is a retired secretary.

Housing Environment: Hazel lives in a Victorian two-bedroom terraced house. The property appears well kept from the outside, with evidence of condensation, rising damp and mould downstairs. The property is double-glazed (all the windows are closed), the heating is on continuously and the ambient temperature is very warm.

Activities of Daily Living (ADLs): Hazel independently manages her medications, dressing and undressing. She mobilises around her home unaided, using furniture to steady herself, occasionally using a stick when her back pain is severe. She can usually get in and out of her recliner chair where she spends most of the day, but tends to sit at the dining table to eat her meals. Hazel rarely uses the kitchen as she cannot stand to prepare foods and struggles to lift a kettle or reach into the cupboards. She can ascend and descend stairs independently using two handrails, but limits this to once a day. She uses the downstairs toilet (she has a freestanding frame) throughout the daytime. It has an extra handrail fitted to assist with sit to stand. Carers assist with showering most days. She can get in and out of bed, however, it can sometimes be a struggle to stand up as it is quite low. She always uses her stick outdoors and rarely goes out alone. She no longer accesses public transport due to her lack of confidence in her mobility and dynamic balance. She manages her own finances and her family have set up direct debits. She uses a landline telephone and does not have a mobile phone or access to the internet.

Carers and Support: Hazel has carers twice daily who assist with meal preparation, providing drinks and snacks. Hazel has frozen meals delivered for her carers to microwave and her daughter does a weekly food shop. Hazel's medication is delivered and she manages this independently. Her family assist with hoovering and mopping the kitchen and bathroom floors. She is socially isolated, experiencing loneliness at times.

Assessment

General Observation: Hazel appears well, alert and orientated to time and place. She has good colour and displays no obvious signs of distress. She appears well perfused, is not clammy or sweaty and has a normal pallor.

Case Study

Clinical Observations

- **Heart rate:** 108 bpm
- **Blood pressure:** 138/74 mmHg (unable to complete standing BP)
- **Blood glucose:** 7.5 mmol
- **Respiratory rate:** 17 breaths per minute
- **Oxygen saturations:** 97% on room air
- **Temperature:** 37.2°C
- **Pupils:** size 3, equal and reactive to light
- **NEWS2 score:** 1
- **Frailty score:** CFS score 6

ABCDE Assessment

Airway: No evidence or signs of airway obstruction. Patent and patient is protecting own airway.

Breathing: Completing full sentences. No evidence of distress or increased work of breathing.

Circulation: Appears well perfused with warm peripheries, capillary refill time three seconds, regular pulse. Skin turgor reduced with no peripheral oedema. ECG shows sinus tachycardia. Normal heart sounds with no added sounds.

Disability: AVPU = A, PEARL = 3 bilaterally, GCS score = 15/15, 4AT score = 0. No evidence of new confusion. FAST-negative, moving all four limbs spontaneously with no new or focal neurological changes. Pain score reported as 0 in sitting.

Exposure: No new abdominal symptoms. No vomiting, but says she regularly feels nauseous which has increased over the last few days. Bowels not opened for three days. No urinary signs. Bowel sounds present throughout, mildly tender on palpation, left iliac fossa and flank. Firmness and slightly dull to percuss. Patient not complaining of any specific new joint or bone pain. No recent history of trauma, no obvious signs of injury, wounds or infection, no shortening, rotation or altered posture.

Holistic Assessment: Hazel is not in significant distress, but functionally it is unsafe for her to remain at home as she is unable to transfer in and out of her chair with carer support. Hazel feels safe at home and wishes to remain there and is happy to receive help and care at home.

Impression: Constipation and dehydration. Possible acute kidney injury.

Treatment Plan: Admission to hospital via ED does not seem clinically indicated or appropriate. A referral to a UCR with a two-hour response time would be best for this patient.

CHAPTER 7   Activities of Daily Living

Introduction

Activities of daily living (ADLs) are the activities we engage in to maintain survival and include the essential skills required to ensure we can manage our basic physical needs (Edemekong et al., 2022). ADLs are comprised of the following areas: mobility and transfers, maintaining personal hygiene needs such as grooming, washing, dressing and managing continence and toileting needs, as well as eating and maintaining nutrition and hydration (Mlinac and Feng, 2016). Although the term ADL is broadly used in health and social care settings to quickly communicate a persons functional status, ADLs can be broken down into two separate categories: basic ADLs (BADLs), those which involve attending to our physical needs; and instrumental ADLs (IADLs), those which involve complex cognitive processes associated with executive functioning and provide us with the skills to enable independent living within the community (Johnson et al., 2007; Marshall et al., 2011; Ong et al., 2021).

Executive functioning can be defined as a series of cognitive processes we use day to day which allow us to complete our daily tasks and are controlled by the frontal lobe of the brain (Dimond, 2013). They can be categorised into two separate domains: organisation and regulation (University of California San Francisco, 2022). Organisation involves skills such as attention, planning and cognitive flexibility. Regulation involves, for example, initiation, emotional regulation and self-awareness. These skills allow us to manage finances, medications, maintain social relationships, complete household tasks, such as laundry and shopping, hold down employment, as well as drive a car or use public transport.

Sudden Onset Immobility

Immobility is one of five recognised frailty syndromes (see Chapter 3: Frailty); sudden onset reduced mobility is a key indicator of clinical frailty. The urgent care presentation of an older person with a sudden onset of reduced mobility should be thoroughly investigated to uncover the potential underlying illness. A person should not be deemed as 'off legs' without an underlying cause for this acute change in their function (see also Chapter 8: Falls). It is possible to have any of these problems without frailty and sometimes there can be a very straightforward explanation for the problem. However, a sudden change in mobility or a fall in an older person with clinical frailty could indicate serious underlying illness (Clegg et al., 2013).

Sudden onset immobility or reduced function adversely affects the quality of life of older people, threatens their independence and personal autonomy and increases both informal and formal carer needs. Inactivity increases the risks of incontinence, pressure ulcers, deep vein thrombosis, osteoporosis, pulmonary embolism, risks of muscular weakness, lowered aerobic capacity and finally leads to poor physical capacity or deconditioning (Wu et al., 2018).

Causes and Symptoms of Immobility

Constipation, and the discomfort associated with constipation, can lead to significant issues with functional mobility (Gandell et al., 2013) as can dehydration (Begum and

Johnson, 2010). Muscle weakness, lethargy and fatigue are common symptoms of both. The older population is up to 30% more likely to develop dehydration and while poor mobility may be a symptom, in Hazel's case, it can also be a cause (Miller, 2015). Acute illness will undoubtedly contribute to a deterioration in the ability to perform ADLs (Covinsky et al., 2003; Sands et al., 2002). Other influencing factors affecting the ability to carry out ADLs, aside from acute illness and hospitalisation, are the side effects of medications and polypharmacy (see Chapter 6: Polypharmacy and Medicines Review) in addition to the person's environment itself (Chu et al., 2020; Farias et al., 2003).

Conducting a Functional Assessment

Functional assessment involves the assessment of a wide range of functions and ADLs. Some of the assessments will rely on patients self-reporting their own abilities or difficulties and other domains will be objectively observed or formally assessed. Gathering collateral history from a patient's family or carers can be an essential part of creating an assessment picture (Fitzpatrick et al., 2020).

There are several validated objective assessment tools that can more formally assess ADLs:

- Katz Index of Independence in Activities of Daily Living (Katz et al., 1963)
- Barthel United Kingdom Index of Activities of Daily Living (Mahoney and Barthel, 1965)
- Modified Barthel Index of Activities of Daily Living (Collin et al., 1988; Shah et al., 1989)
- Nottingham Extended Activities of Daily Living Scale (University of Nottingham, 2007).

Specific Functional Assessments

Assessment of Sitting Balance

To assess this, generally observe the following:

- Does the patient appear comfortable sat in their chair?
- Are they slumped or sitting to one side?
- Are they able to pick up objects around their chair reaching outside of their base of support in sitting?
- How does their balance change if they close their eyes?
- Are they able to lift one or both feet off the floor independently?
- Are they able to 'scoot' their buttocks forward in the chair independently?

The function in sitting test (FIST) will offer a more detailed and structured assessment of sitting balance, particularly useful in patients with neurological conditions such as stroke (Gorman et al., 2010; Gorman et al., 2014a; Gorman et al., 2014b).

CHAPTER 7 Activities of Daily Living

Sit-to-Stand Objective Assessment

Sit-to-stand (STS) and stand-to-sit (SIT) transfers are incredibly important movements, STS being the most frequently occurring movement – an essential precursor to independent walking (Galli et al., 2008). It involves moving the body's centre of mass forward out of the sitting base of support. When it is above the feet in contact with the floor you will be able to lift your buttocks off the seat without loss of balance (Lomaglio and Eng, 2005). Biomechanically it is quite a challenging task, as the body moves from a static stable position (seated), through an unstable dynamic phase, through to a semi-stable phase in standing (Hughes, 1996). Performing this movement successfully demands strength, coordination, motor control and momentum.

The height of the seat is a crucial factor to be able to STS. Less exertion is needed to rise from a chair with a higher seat height. A chair that is too high may be easier to STS from due to the reduced effort and distance required in the task, but stability will be significantly compromised in sitting. The knees should never be above the hips in sitting, for pelvic posture, hip strength and flexibility, but also for circulatory and lymphatic drainage reasons. It is important to assess the posture the chair is stuck in and to determine whether the mechanism is broken or has moved recently. This could be a contributory, yet reversible, factor. An occupational therapy assessment would always be recommended if seating is considered an issue which is affecting function.

If a patient can STS independently, you would observe the following factors:

- Are they able to rise from the chair or toilet using no arms, one arm or do they use both?
- Observe the height and type of chair. Are they using any specialist seating or equipment?
- Do they take several attempts to build the momentum to stand or rock themselves back and forth?
- How many attempts are required to successfully stand up from seated?
- Did they pull themselves up using a walking frame, rail or other object? (This may be unsafe if not appropriately fixed and could cause injuries.)
- How much effort and exertion can you observe in the patient? Was this subjectively easy or extremely difficult?
- How do they sit back down into the chair? Do they lower themselves in a controlled way or flop down suddenly and unsafely?

Correct assessment of STS is important. You must take into consideration the patient's strength, any pain or discomfort, ability to follow instructions, motivation and seating. Ask the patient how they normally rise from seated: do they have assistance, use handling belts with carers or lifting equipment? Only attempt to assess a person up to their normal level of ability and proceed with assessing transfers once you are satisfied it is safe to continue.

Toileting

All the discussion above regarding STS can be applied to sitting down and standing up from a toilet or commode. While the principles are the same, heights and arms are often different, so you must not assume that a person who can STS comfortably from an armchair is able to do so from a toilet seat. Do they require a rail to pull up on? Sinks and radiators are often used, and damaged, when patients pull up their body weight.

Sitting and standing from toilet furniture is one thing, however the joint range of movement, coordination and strength to be able to wipe and clean oneself after using the toilet is also important to consider. This is often overlooked in acute upper limb injuries, for example, wrist fracture. Long handle sponges and other aids and adaptations may be recommended by an occupational therapist for patients struggling in maintaining personal hygiene. For more detailed assessments of washing, dressing and bathing, you would refer the patient for specialist assessment by an occupational therapist.

Static and Dynamic Balance

Balance is crucial for many ADLs and refers to the ability to maintain your line of gravity, within your base of support. The somatosensory, visual and vestibular systems all work harmoniously to contribute to an individual being able to maintain balance independently. Static balance is the ability to maintain postural stability when the body is at rest (Bannister, 1969). Dynamic balance is the ability to maintain postural stability when the body is moving, for example walking, standing up or reaching for an object (O'Sullivan and Portney, 2014). There are several simple balance tests that may help in uncovering a problem with balance including the Romberg test, four stage balance test and the functional reach test.

Gait and Mobility

Physical movement is a basic human need (Rantanen, 2013). A complex interplay between cardiorespiratory, nervous and musculoskeletal systems contribute to our ability to walk. Figure 7.1 illustrates the two phases of walking, with seven components. During the stance phase, weight shifts onto a single limb, as the opposite limb is in swing phase.

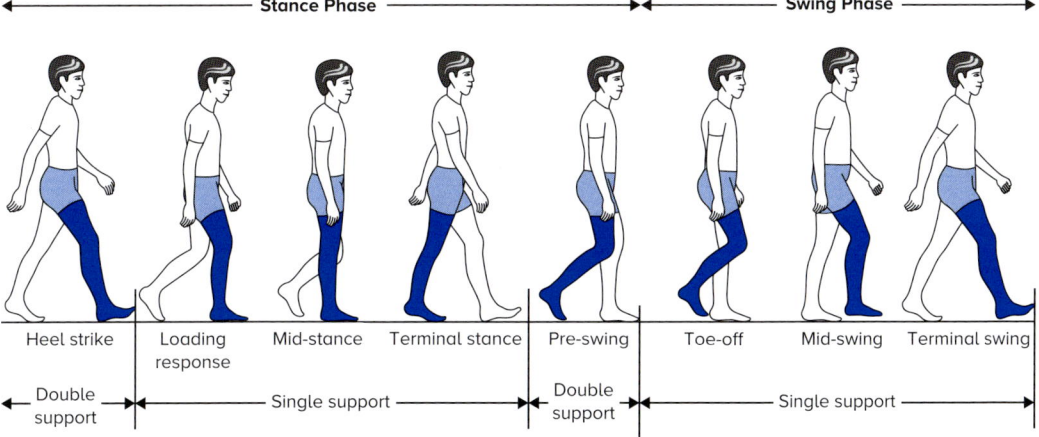

Figure 7.1 The gait cycle.
Source: Maetzler et al. (2016). Gait disorders in adults and the elderly: A clinical guide. Licensed under CC BY 4.0. https://creativecommons.org/licenses/by/4.0/

CHAPTER 7 Activities of Daily Living

General observation of walking should look for any obvious neurological deficit, abnormal muscle tone or sensation in lower limbs, any joint deformities or abnormal postures. You should consider:

- How does the patient begin walking?
- Are they hesitating or taking multiple attempts to begin?
- What is the step height and is it equal for both feet?
- Are steps symmetrical?
- Is the patient deviating from a planned path during the journey to grab hold of something for stability?
- What is happening in the trunk, is there rotation and adequate arm swing?
- Is the patient able to stop when intended?
- Are they able to change direction or turn round safely?
- Are they becoming noticeably short of breath during the assessment requiring a rest?
- How far is the patient able to walk?
- Is distance limited by breathlessness, pain or weakness?

Some common ways gait patterns can be described is included in Table 7.1:

Table 7.1 Gait patterns.

Gait	Description
Antalgic gait	An adopted gait pattern often described as limping. Adopted to avoid weight-bearing through painful joints and structures.
Ataxic gait	Unsteady or uncoordinated gait pattern with a wide base of support, high steps or slapping feet. Pathological causes may include cerebellar pathologies or long-term alcohol dependence.
Parkinsonian gait	Commonly seen in Parkinson's disease, rigid postures, narrow base of support, reduced arm swing, forward flexed posture.
Festinating gait	Rapid small steps, speeding up involuntarily, a forward lean in the trunk.
Hemiplegic gait	Hip flexed and the leg is circumducted due to foot drop.
High step/neuropathic gait	The leg is lifted high in the air, an exaggerated step clearing the ground.
Waddling gait	Exaggerated lateral trunk movements from side to side, often seen in osteoarthritis.
Trendelenburg gait	A drooping of the pelvis, on the opposite side to weak or paralysed hip abductor muscles.
Diplegic/scissoring gait	Associated with spasticity in both lower limbs. Knees and hips pressed together, often legs may cross over.

Specific Functional Assessments

There are several validated objective assessment tools that can more formally assess walking:

- TUGT (Podsiadlo and Richardson, 1991)
- Tinetti Gait and Balance Instrument (Tinetti, 1986)
- Dynamic Gait Index (Shumway-Cook and Woollacott, 1995)
- POMA (Performance-oriented Mobility Assessment) (Tinetti, 1986)
- Elderly Mobility Scale (EMS) (Smith, 1994).

Gait Speed Test

The gait speed test simply measures the time it takes for a person to walk 4 metres. Four metres was suggested as a sensible distance, as it is the estimated average length of a person's living room in the UK. If a person takes longer than 5 seconds to walk 4 metres then this predicts future disability (Abellan Van Kan et al., 2009).

Slow walking speed has good sensitivity but only moderate specificity for identifying frailty. For example, only one in three older people (over 75 years) with slow walking speed is living with frailty (Abellan Van Kan et al., 2009). Regardless of this, a person with a slower walking speed must be screened for frailty and assessed with this in mind. The gait speed test is not diagnostic and should not give the patient a label, but it can be particularly useful in suggesting or predicting the likelihood of underlying frailty needing further assessment. The gait speed test is one example of a functional assessment. There are other appropriate tests depending upon the setting.

Upper Limb Function

Age-related changes in the shoulder joint can impair range of motion (ROM). Many older patients may be unaware of shoulder limitations since dysfunction develops insidiously and without pain. Lack of shoulder mobility can impede a person's ability to drive, dress and reach items in a wardrobe or kitchen cupboard. Long-term problems may result in muscle weakness, reduced endurance, chronic pain, sleep disturbance and reduced ROM. This is also a prediction of reduced grip strength and difficulty in performing ADLs. A simple test is to inquire about pain and observe shoulder ROM.

Normal hand function may be impaired by arthritis, neurological problems, vascular disease or trauma. The ability to grasp and pinch are needed for dressing, grooming, toileting and feeding. Hand and finger dexterity can be evaluated by asking the patient to pick up small objects (coins, eating utensils or cup) from a flat surface. Another measure is grasp strength: the patient is asked to squeeze two of the examiner's fingers with each hand. Pinch strength can be assessed by having the patient firmly hold a sheet of paper between the thumb and index finger, while the clinician tries to pull it out. If the patient has difficulty with this test, physiotherapy or occupational therapy assessment will be useful.

Sarcopenia is associated with increased adverse outcomes including falls, functional decline, frailty and mortality. Hand grip strength is used to diagnose both

CHAPTER 7 Activities of Daily Living

sarcopenia and frailty and can predict not only overall strength and health, but also risk of cardiovascular disease. As you age, the stronger your grip, the more likely you are to survive diseases like cancer (Zhuang et al., 2020). Maintaining muscle mass and, as part of that, grip strength are important for mobility and strength.

Walking Aids

Walking Stick

The stick is held in the opposite hand to the weaker leg. This ensures it helps take the weight off the weaker, or more painful, leg. If it is held on the same side it encourages the patient to lean over to that side and take more weight onto the affected leg. The stick goes forward with, and is placed level with, the affected leg. It is not safe for a stick to be placed too far forward or left behind.

Walking sticks are used to provide support, confidence and stability. They are not designed to take the full weight from a leg or have too much weight put through them. If a patient appears to be leaning very heavily through a stick, it may be worth considering another aid. Problems with the upper limb may limit or restrict the choice of upper limb to hold the stick – this must be considered.

Frames

Always check the general condition of the frame. If the frame has wheels it is meant to be pushed (many patients do not do this, they lift and place). If the frame does not have wheels on it is meant to be lifted and placed. These frames are more stable, but less mobile.

The frame is pushed just past the end of the feet, then the affected leg is stepped into the frame level with the back legs of the frame. The other leg is then stepped to the same level.

If feet are placed too far forward into the frame this creates an increased risk of the patient falling backwards. If patients step through and each foot is placed past the other then this is fine as it mimics a more normal gait pattern, however they need to keep the frame moving.

Stairs

The Royal Society for the Prevention of Accidents recognised stair safety as a considerable hazard to the UK population and has deemed falls on the stairs to be 'a hidden killer' which results in the loss of over 700 lives in England every year and hospitalises 43,000 people (Garrett et al., 2021).

Attention should be paid to additional underlying factors, for example, functional decline in older adults due to loss of muscle strength, stamina, polypharmacy and visual decline contribute to poor mobility and disability, resulting in an inability or difficulty in safely navigating stairs (Elliot et al., 2015; Hamel et al., 2005; Heasley et al., 2004; Startzell et al., 2000; Templer, 1994). Poor grip strength when pulling up on the stair rail, not putting the foot fully on the stair tread, poor footwear and thread bear or confusing carpet patterns are other influences that will result in falls, injuries and potential death (Templer, 1994).

The design and the style of staircases can influence these factors and play a significant role. For example, the impact of stair risers on fatigue levels, surface type, shallow tread depth and nosing type are all evident at various levels in causing accidents.

It is therefore imperative that consideration is given to the multiple elements that contribute to falls on the stairs. Research has shown that providing home modifications such as stair rails and balustrades can be a means of reducing injuries (Keall et al., 2015). Highlighting issues and concerns to emergency departments (EDs) and community urgent care/rapid response services, housing trusts and agencies such as Age Concern, Care and Repair England and the local authority could help in ensuring risks are addressed early. Referring to community falls and therapy services will further support improving and maintaining functional performance and can reduce hazards that contribute to trips and falls.

Handrails

Handrails are used to provide stability and support. They are not safe to be used as 'parallel bars' to drag or pull oneself up the stairs. Have a look at the patient's knuckles – how tight are they gripping and pulling up on the handrail? Also, how far in front are their hands being placed? If it is more than one full step in front or a comfortable length, it may be that they are relying too much on their upper limbs – this is not a safe way to climb the stairs.

Additionally, it is important handrails are held with a full grip, not one or two fingers or just an elbow or a fist. If a patient requires one or two handrails on the stairs, it must be reinforced to them that this always applies and it is not safe to carry anything up or down the stairs.

The Environment

Cold, damp and inadequately insulated homes due to poor energy efficiency and low quality heating mostly affects those from deprived socioeconomic backgrounds and those on low incomes (Local Government Association, 2014). Cold temperatures and poorly heated homes are associated with poorer health outcomes such as respiratory diseases, exacerbated diabetes, increased risk of frailty, stroke, increased levels of anxiety and depression, increased risk of falls and accidents for older people and, at worse, death (Marmot Review Team, 2011). Temperatures below the recommended 18°C can exacerbate cardiovascular issues, circulatory problems and leg ulcers (Public Health England, 2014).

Morbidity and mortality due to heat disproportionately affects older people, regardless of whether there is obvious disease or not. This is due to compromised cardiovascular and thermoregulatory reactions which occur during the ageing process (Kenney, et al., 2014). Increased temperatures place considerable pressure on the cardiovascular system, the body's defence mechanisms such as sweating and can lead to cardiovascular strain and hospitalisation through heat exhaustion and heat stroke (Gagnon, et al., 2016).

Carbon monoxide from faulty gas appliances and boilers are of a specific risk to health, particularly in homes that have not been regularly serviced and with appliances that are old and in need of replacing. Chronic low-level exposure to carbon monoxide in indoor air can lead to significant adverse effects, such as certain neurological conditions (Croxford et al., 2008).

Residents who live in properties that experience damp and mould are at increased risk of developing respiratory infections and conditions such as aspergillosis, asthma and allergic rhinitis (Jaakkola et al., 2013; Quansah et al., 2012). Skin conditions such as eczema and certain allergies may be exacerbated. The three factors that contribute to the build-up of condensation are poor ventilation, high humidity and low temperature of walls and surfaces. Although some people are more sensitive to the effects of mould than others, such as those with defective immune systems, those with pre-existing respiratory conditions and older people are most at risk.

Floor covering can have a detrimental impact on health (Becher et al., 2018). While they offer benefits such as thermal comfort, a sense of safety, noise reduction and cushioning underfoot, carpeting that is old and dirty can harbour dust mites, toxic chemicals and allergens (Vaughan and Platts-Mills, 2000). Respiratory, haematological and neurological illnesses, can result from exposure to these agents (Roberts and Dickey, 1995). Rugs that are a known trip hazard have the same impact as carpet (Becher et al., 2018).

Motivation

A barrier to performing a task may be physical, it may be environmental or it may be due to a lack of motivation to perform it. This must be considered within your assessment of a patient, without placing your own opinions or ideas upon the person. They may have 'lost' motivation for something, and may wish to regain it, or it may be something they have no interest in being independent in. Try and explore the barrier to a task and if there are ways forward.

A patient may be avoiding washing and dressing in clean clothes daily because it is exhausting, they struggle with the dexterity and physical demands of the task or they cannot access the bathing facilities comfortably. Try to encourage very small manageable goals for change to increase success and in turn fuel further motivation. Offer practical solutions that may make the task more manageable to increase the appetite for change. Health promotion is vital at every opportunity. This could be the moment your patient feels empowered.

Insight and Risk

A lack of insight, or a lack of risk assessment, is different to a lack in motivation. An individual who over or underestimates their own physical or functional ability has the potential for harm. If an older person assumes they cannot manage a task, they will not try. They may become dependent on support they do not always need, for example meal and drink preparation. It is important to be clear with patients that they should maintain their independence and actively function to their full potential. Failure to do this can result in more rapid decline and deconditioning. On the opposing side, attempting a task that requires a higher level of physical strength or balance than they possess may result in injury. For example, an older person with reduced core strength trying to lift a heavy object is likely to injure themselves. It is important to gauge whether a patient has good and accurate insight into their own levels of ability, so they set both achievable and safe functional goals for themselves.

Conclusion

It is essential to make every contact count, and recognition of even subtle signs of poor ADL performance should be escalated with the MDT admission avoidance service, if available, or the GP as soon as possible to ensure prompt assessment and investigation takes place, particularly in those situations where hospital admission is not warranted. It is estimated that one-third of older adults will experience a decline in ADL function following a hospital admission, with those over the age of 85 experiencing the most significant loss in function (Boltz et al., 2012). Therefore, these functional assessments form a crucial component of the overall assessment of the older person in their home environment.

Questions

1. Consider this chapter's content and apply what you have learnt to a recent patient or family member.

2. Thinking about this person, what frailty syndromes or conditions can you identify?

3. How do the theories of ageing affect the presentations described in this chapter?

References

Abellan Van Kan G, et al. (2009). Gait speed at usual pace as a predictor of adverse outcomes in community-dwelling older people an International Academy on Nutrition and Aging (IANA) Task Force. *Journal of Nutrition, Health and Aging*, 13(9): 881–889.

Bannister R (1969). *Brain's Clinical Neurology* (3rd edition). New York: Oxford University Press.

Becher R et al. (2018). Do carpets impair indoor air quality and cause adverse health outcomes: a review. *International Journal of Environmental Research and Public Health*, 15(2): 184.

Begum MN, Johnson CS (2010). A review of the literature on dehydration in the institutionalized elderly. *Clinical Nutrition ESPEN*, 5(1): 47–53.

Boltz M, Resnick B, Galik E (2012). Interventions to prevent functional decline in the acute care setting. In *Evidence-based Geriatric Nursing Protocols for Best Practice* (4th edition), Boltz et al. (eds.). New York: Springer Publishing Company: 104–121.

CHAPTER 7   Activities of Daily Living

Centre for Ageing Better (2015). Home and dry. The need for decent homes in later life. Available at: https://ageing-better.org.uk/resources/home-and-dry-need-decent-homes-later-life [accessed 6th August 2024].

Chu NM, et al. (2020). Functional independence, access to kidney transplantation and waitlist mortality. *Nephrology Dialysis Transplantation*, 35(5): 870–877.

Clegg A, et al. (2013). Frailty in elderly people. *The Lancet*, 381(9868): 752–762.

Collin C, et al. (1988). The Barthel ADL Index: A reliability study. *International Disability Studies*, 10(2): 61–63.

Covinsky KE, et al. (2003). Loss of independence in activities of daily living in older adults hospitalized with medical illnesses: increased vulnerability with age. *Journal of the American Geriatrics Society*, 51(4): 451–458.

Croxford B, Leonardi G, Kreis I (2008). Self-reported neurological symptoms in relation to CO emissions due to problem gas appliance installations in London: a cross-sectional survey. *Environmental Health*, 7: 34.

Dimond A (2013). Executive functions. *Annual Review of Psychology*, 64: 135–168.

Edemekong PF, et al. (2022). Activities of daily living. In *StatPearls* (Internet). Treasure Island: StatPearls Publishing.

Elliott DB, et al. (2015). Analysis of lower limb movement to determine the effect of manipulating the appearance of stairs to improve safety: a linked series of laboratory-based, repeated measures studies. *Public Health Research*, 3(8).

Farias, ST, et al. (2003). The relationship between neuropsychological performance and daily functioning in individuals with Alzheimer's disease: ecological validity of neuropsychological tests. *Archives of Clinical Neuropsychology*, 18(6): 655–672.

Fitzpatrick D, et al. (2020). The collateral history: an overlooked core clinical skill. *European Geriatric Medicine*, 11(6): 1003–1007.

Gagnon D, et al. (2016). Cardiac and thermal strain of elderly adults exposed to extreme heat and humidity with and without electric fan use. *Journal of the American Medical Association*, 316: 989–991.

Galli M, et al. (2008). Quantitative analysis of sit to stand movement: experimental set-up definition and application to healthy and hemiplegic adults. *Gait Posture*, 28(1): 80–85.

Gandell D, et al. (2013). Treatment of constipation in older people. *Canadian Medical Association Journal*, 185(8): 663–670.

Garrett H, et al. (2021). The cost of poor housing. BRE Group. Available at: https://files.bregroup.com/research/BRE_Report_the_cost_of_poor_housing_2021.pdf [accessed 30th August 2024].

Gorman SL, et al. (2010). Development and validation of the function in sitting test in adults with acute stroke. *Journal of Neurologic Physical Therapy*, 34(3): 150–160.

Gorman SL, et al. (2014a). Examining the function in sitting test for validity. Responsiveness, and minimally clinically important difference in inpatient rehabilitation. *Archives of Physical Medicine and Rehabilitation*, 95(12): 2304–2311.

Gorman SL, Rivera M, McCarthy L (2014b). Reliability of the function in sitting test (FIST). *Rehabilitation Research and Practice*, 2014: 593280.

Hamel KA, et al. (2005). Foot clearance during stair descent: effects of age and illumination. *Gait Posture*, 21(2): 135–140.

Heasley K, et al. (2004). Stepping up to a new level: effects of blurring vision in the elderly. *Investigative Ophthalmology Visual Science*, 45(7): 2122–2128.

Hughes MA, Myers BS, Schenkman ML (1996). The role of strength in rising from a chair in the functionally impaired elderly. *Journal of Biomechanics*, 29(12): 1509–1513.

Jaakkola MS, et al. (2013). Association of indoor dampness and moulds with rhinitis risk: a systematic review and meta-analysis. *Journal of Allergy and Clinical Immunology*, 132(5): 1099–1110.

References

Johnson JK, Lui LY, Yaffe K (2007). Executive function, more than global cognition, predicts functional decline and mortality in elderly women. *The Journals of Gerontology Series A Biological Sciences and Medical Sciences*, 62(10): 1134–1141.

Katz et al. (1963). Studies of illness in the aged: The Index of ADL: A Standardized Measure of Biological and Psychosocial Function. *JAMA*, 185(12): 914–919.

Keall MD, Pierse N, Howden-Chapman P (2015). Home modifications to reduce injuries from falls in the Home Injury Prevention Intervention (HIPI) study: a cluster-randomised controlled trial. *The Lancet*, 385(9964): 231–238.

Kenney WL, Craighead DH, Alexander LM (2014). Heat waves, aging, and human cardiovascular health. *Medical Science and Sports Exercise*, 46(10): 1891–1899.

Local Government Association (2014). Healthy homes, healthy lives. London. Available at: https://www.local.gov.uk/publications/healthy-homes-healthy-lives [accessed 6th August 2024].

Lomaglio MJ, Eng JJ (2005). Muscle strength and weight-bearing symmetry relate to sit-to-stand performance in individuals with stroke. *Gait Posture*, 22(2): 126–131.

Mahoney FI and Barthel DW (1965). Functional evaluation: The Barthel Index. *Maryland Sate Medical Journal*, 14: 61–65.

Marmot Review Team (2011). The health impacts of cold homes and fuel poverty. Available at: https://www.instituteofhealthequity.org/resources-reports/the-health-impacts-of-cold-homes-and-fuel-poverty/the-health-impacts-of-cold-homes-and-fuel-poverty.pdf [accessed 6th August 2024].

Marshall GA, et al. (2011). Alzheimer's disease neuroimaging initiative. Executive function and instrumental activities of daily living in mild cognitive impairment and Alzheimer's disease. *Alzheimer's and Dementia*, 7(3): 300–308.

Miller HJ (2015). Dehydration in the older adult. *Journal of Gerontological Nursing*, 41(9): 8–13.

Mlinac ME and Feng MC (2016). Assessment of activities of daily living, self-care, and independence. *Archives of Clinical Neuropsychology*, 31(6): 506–516.

Office for National Statistics (2022). Emergency hospital admissions due to falls in people aged 65–79. Public Health Profiles. Available at: https://www.gov.uk/government/publications/falls-applying-all-our-health/falls-applying-all-our-health [accessed 6th August 2024].

Ong M, et al. (2021). Social frailty and executive function: association with geriatric syndromes, life space and quality of life in healthy community-dwelling older adults. *Journal of Frailty and Aging*, 11(2): 206–213.

O'Sullivan SB, Portney LG (2014). *Physical Rehabilitation* (6th edition). Philadelphia: FA Davis.

Pauls J (2011). Perception and cognition. Paper presented at the International Conference on Stairway Usability and Safety, June 9–10, 2011, Toronto, Canada.

Podsiadlo D and Richardson S (1991). Timed 'Up & Go': A test of basic functional mobility for frail elderly persons. *Journal of the American Geriatrics Society*, 39(2): 142–148.

Public Health England (2014). Minimum home temperature thresholds for health in winter – A systematic literature review. Available at: https://assets.publishing.service.gov.uk/media/5c5986f8ed915d045f3778a9/Min_temp_threshold_for_homes_in_winter.pdf [accessed 14th October 2024].

Quansah R, et al. (2012). Residential dampness and moulds and the risk of developing asthma: a systematic review and meta-analysis. *Public Library of Science One*, 7(11): e47526.

Rantanen T (2013). Promoting mobility in older people. *Journal of Preventive Medicine and Public Health*, 46(Suppl 1): S50–54.

Roberts JW, Dickey P (1995). Exposure of children to pollutants in house dust and indoor air. *Reviews of Environmental Contamination and Toxicology*, 143: 59–78.

Royal College of Physicians (2011). NHS services for falls and fractures in older people are inadequate, finds national clinical audit. Available at: https://www.rcp.ac.uk/news-and-media/

news-and-opinion/nhs-services-for-falls-and-fractures-in-older-people-are-inadequate-finds-national-clinical-audit/ [accessed 6th August 2024].

Sands L, et al. (2002). The effects of acute illness on ADL decline over 1 year in frail older adults with and without cognitive impairment. *The Journals of Gerontology Series A: Biological Sciences and Medical Sciences*, 57(7): M449–M454.

Shah S, Vanclay F and Cooper B (1989). Improving the sensitivity of the Barthel Index for stroke rehabilitation. *Journal of Clinical Epidemiology*, 42(8): 703–709.

Shumway-Cook A and Woollacott M (1995). The Dynamic Gait Index: A clinical measure of functional mobility for frail elderly persons. *Journal of the American Physical Therapy Association*, 75(6): 519–528.

Smith R (1994). Validation and reliability of the Elderly Mobility *Scale. Physiotherapy*, 80(12): 744–747.

Startzell JK, et al. (2000). Stair negotiation in older people: a review. *Journal of the American Geriatric Society*, 48(5): 567–580.

Templer JA (1994). *The Staircase: Studies of hazards, falls and safer design*. Cambridge: MIT Press.

Tinetti ME (1986). Performance-oriented assessment of mobility problems in elderly patients. *Journal of the American Geriatrics Society*, 34(2): 119–126.

Tinetti ME, et al. (2014). Shared risk factors for falls, incontinence, and functional dependence. In *British Geriatrics Society Best Practice Guide*. London: British Geriatric Society.

University of California San Francisco (2022). Weill Institute for Neurosciences, Memory and Aging centre. Available at: https://memory.ucsf.edu/symptoms/executive-functions [accessed 6th August 2024].

University of Nottingham (2007). Nottingham Extended ADL Scale. Available at: https://www.nottingham.ac.uk/medicine/documents/published-assessments/neadl.pdf [accessed 14th October 2024].

Vaughan JW, Platts-Mills TA (2000). New approaches to environmental control. *Clinical Reviews in Allergy and Immunology*, 18(3): 325–339.

Wu X, et al. (2018). The association between major complications of immobility during hospitalization and quality of life among bedridden patients: a 3 month prospective multi-center study. *PLoS One*, 13(10): e0205729.

Zhuang CL, et al. (2020). Associations of low handgrip strength with cancer mortality: a multicentre observational study. *The Journal of Cachexia, Sarcopenia and Muscle*, 11(6): 1476–1486.

Chapter 8

Falls

Carol Robertson

Learning Points

By the end of this chapter, you will:

- Understand the impact of falls on the patient, care providers and the health service
- Recognise intrinsic and extrinsic causes of falls
- Appreciate the vital role of a holistic approach, referrals and falls prevention
- Understand the importance of asking 'why?'.

Case Study

Background: You are a clinician working within the call centre of an ambulance service undertaking remote triage. At 07:30 the longest waiting call is for an 83-year-old woman, called Ophelia, who has fallen. The electronic notepad states that the caller, Fred (her husband), has advised that it is a non-injury fall but Ophelia is unable to get up. You call the number back, introduce yourself and ask if you can speak with the patient.

Presenting Complaint: An 83-year-old woman has fallen and is still on the floor.

History of Presenting Complaint: Ophelia informs you that she 'tripped' over a rug walking from the bathroom to her bedroom. She and Fred are due to go out with their son later. She says that she does not have the strength or flexibility to get up and Fred, who uses a walking stick, is unable to help her. She says she is not hurt (except her pride) and she is usually so careful, but today she was rushing. She has been on the floor since around 06:50 so feels like she is starting to 'seize up'.

You enquire about what position she is in and how she fell. She informs you that she went onto her knees and then put her hands out, which stopped any impact to her head or chest. She was face down but has managed to turn over and Fred has popped some pillows under her head. You ask if she has sustained any injuries and she informs you that she does not have any pain. You probe further about specific regions with particular focus on her cervical spine, torso, head, hip and pelvis; she confirms nothing hurts and she is currently moving her head, neck and all her limbs as normal. You also question pre-syncopal and syncopal symptoms, but she denies having any. She tells you that she has not fallen previously.

Past Medical History: Arthritis (knees and shoulders), hypertension and diverticulosis.

Allergies: No known drug allergies.

Drug History: Amlodipine (10 mg once daily), paracetamol (1 g up to four times daily).

Social History: Ophelia lives with her husband Fred, completes all her own personal ADLs, including cooking, washing and housework, but it is getting more difficult. They go shopping weekly, usually with one of their children to help push Fred in his wheelchair.

Remote Assessment

Airway: Ophelia can talk freely to you over the phone.

Breathing: She is speaking in full sentences and you can hear a normal breathing pattern during your conversation.

Circulation: Ophelia tells you that Fred says her facial colour is normal and her lips and fingers are normal. She does not have any palpitations and did not experience any chest pain or shortness of breath pre or post fall.

Disabilities: She is not diabetic and Fred has given her a slice of toast and cup of tea while she is on the floor. Further probing elicits Ophelia to be FAST-negative and to have a GCS score of 15/15. She has no dizziness, nausea or vomiting. Ophelia tells you her bowel and bladder activity has been normal over the last few days.

Exposure: Ophelia tells you she is warm enough as the heating is on and Fred has given her a blanket.

Frailty: CFS score 4

Cognition: 4AT – 0. There is no confusion and she is orientated to place, person and time.

Important Considerations: From a protocol approach of sustaining life, major trauma must be excluded; this was determined from the history of the fall, the absence of pain or injuries following the specific questions regarding cervical spine, spine, head, torso and pelvic region. The next priority is to exclude significant illness such as cardiac related syncopal event, stroke or loss of consciousness. Furthermore, was it a fall?

Initial Impression: Non-syncopal fall due to an extrinsic factor (rug), but further questioning is required as it is important to gain a collateral history of events.

Initial Plan: Following a full assessment and the information provided (confirmed by Fred) you are assured that this was a non-syncopal fall. The next consideration is how to get Ophelia from the floor safely. Ophelia is unable to get herself up and Fred cannot assist. You are aware of a falls lifting service who can attend within a suitable timeframe, so you explain to her what this entails. Ophelia agrees to the service. While she awaits this resource you advise her to keep moving to prevent pressure areas, encourage fluids, take her prescribed medications and required analgesia (if safe to do so, for example, she has the ability to sit upright enough to eat and drink) while waiting. Lastly, you advise her to call 999 should she deteriorate, or experience any further issues while waiting, so she can be reassessed.

Following the attendance of the 'falls lifting service', they contact you to inform you that Ophelia has been assisted from the floor using their equipment, and they confirm she has no injuries. You ask if Ophelia experienced any light-headedness or similar on being assisted, they confirm she did not. The falls lifting team will complete a falls prevention assessment while there and discuss further referrals such as occupational therapists or medications team referral to prevent further falls. Finally, you request Ophelia informs her GP of her fall to enable this event to be logged. You also advise her to check for red areas which have been in contact with the floor in case of any developing pressure areas.

Introduction

A fall can be defined as an incident which causes an individual to inadvertently be on the ground and which is not due to a major intrinsic event (for example, stroke) or a substantial hazard (the Office for Health Improvement and Disparities (OHID), 2022). Anyone can fall – it is an unwelcome, but common consequence of the human anatomy and, unfortunately, as we age, falling – although not normal or acceptable – is more common (OHID, 2022). Approximately a third of people over 65 and half of those over 80 will fall at least once per year (Ganz and Latham, 2020; NICE, 2019; NHS, 2021a). Those at high risk of further falls include individuals who require assistance with their ADLs and those who have experienced a previous fall and/or a recent hospital stay (Clemson et al., 2023; OHID, 2022). However, it is vital that age is not blamed for the cause of a fall. It is not 'just a fall' and a full account and understanding of the individual's circumstances needs to be explored.

Falls are a recognised frailty syndrome; they are often a predictable consequence of altered gait and physical motion. The impact to the individual can be devastating, from loss of confidence to disability requiring full-time care and even mortality (OHID, 2022). Falls are usually multifactorial and are frequently associated with risk factors, of which there are over 400. The sum of an individual's risk factors suggest a correlation with the number of falls (National Institute for Health and Care Excellence (NICE) (2017).

Assessing an Older Person Who Has Fallen (Remotely or Face-to-Face)

Assessing an older person who has fallen needs to be thorough as it is often the result of something else, for example, acute illness (Clegg et al., 2013). Many older people do not present with typical symptoms of illness, for example, the cough and low oxygen saturations often seen in COVID, rather than an unexplained fall, which is often secondary to the COVID-19 infection (Zazzara et al., 2021). Also, if an older person has managed to walk with their wheeled walking frame for several years without incident, ask – "what has changed today?" You need to explore if there has been a gradual or sudden deterioration in their function or care needs because a sudden deterioration suggests something underlying (Clegg et al., 2013).

Assessing an older person is complex and you may need to explore many aspects of their daily routine to discover the cause or catalyst of the fall. Once major trauma and critical reversible illness has been ruled out, the holistic approach for older people is the most suitable. This not only encompasses their medical requirements, but also their cognition (including capacity), social needs, function and advance care plans. Only with this added information can you understand what has changed today and how best to address it and agree a safe plan. Taking time to understand an individual's baseline will assist with this. Collating this information and identifying the patient's frailty score (assessed on their baseline two weeks previously) will help to determine any acute issues.

Your assessment should determine the type and cause of the fall such as pre-syncopal, syncopal or non-syncopal and involving intrinsic or extrinsic factors considering the validity of the patient's and/or witnesses' recollections. It is not unusual to 'fill in the blanks'. Syncope is defined as:

> 'transient loss of consciousness due to cerebral hypoperfusion, characterised by a rapid onset, short duration and spontaneous complete recovery'
>
> (NICE, 2023a).

A syncope can have numerous triggers, including life-threatening and benign events. However, no cause is determined in a third of episodes (British Medical Journal (BMJ), 2022a). Causes can include cardiac (MI), reflex (vasovagal syndrome, carotid sinus syndrome); orthostatic (dysautonomia, hypovolaemia), neurological, anatomical, metabolic or psychiatric (BMJ, 2022a).

Pre-syncope, also referred to as near-syncope, often has various meanings to diverse providers but signifies near fainting that can last for seconds to minutes (Whitledge et al., 2023). It arises when an individual almost loses consciousness, usually due to a reduction in oxygenated blood flow to the brain (Newcastle Hospitals NHS Foundation Trust, 2020). It is often referred to as light-headedness, vertigo, wooziness, giddiness or a feeling of being drunk (Woodford, 2022; Newcastle Hospitals NHS Foundation Trust, 2020).

Consider the position the patient is in on the floor: does anything suggest that an individual may have had a syncopal event rather than fallen? An important factor to consider is where their hands are. Figure 8.1 demonstrates upper limb positions. Does the information provided suggest that the patient was able to put their hands out to prevent hitting their face or head? Do they have any head or facial injuries suggesting they could not protect themselves (possible pre-syncopal or syncopal fall). Or are there any upper limb injuries which suggests they were able to put their arms out to break their fall (non-syncopal or pre-syncopal). If assessing remotely, it is important to gain this information and formulate a 'picture' of how the fall happened and what injuries they may have sustained.

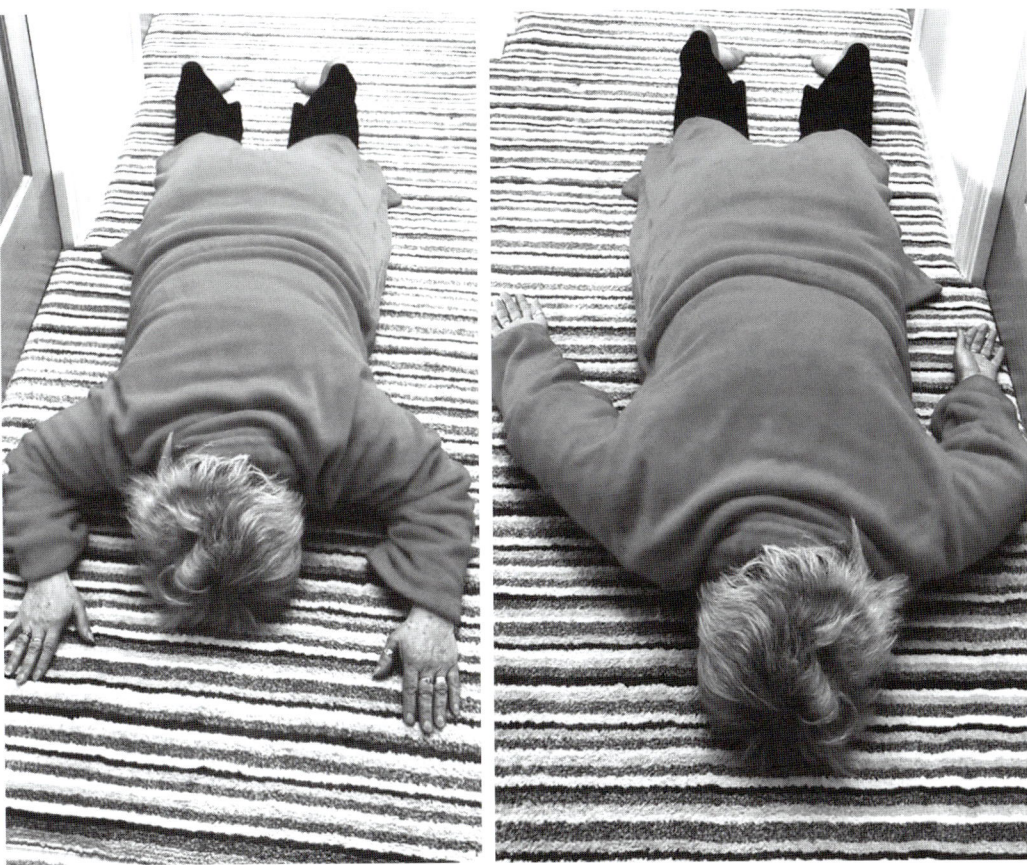

Figure 8.1 Hand position to indicate fall or syncopal event.
Source: Photographs © Carol Robertson.

Furthermore, assessing the length of time the patient may have been on the floor is also important. Clues may include, are they wearing suitable clothing for the time of day? Have you noticed the presence of any incontinence? Does the environment match with the information provided? Are the curtains opened? Most people do not want to give false information, but it is easy for both the patient, relative, carer and/or clinician to fill in the gaps and make assumptions about what could have happened. Other questions to ask or observe are: has the bed been slept in? Are there signs of the patient having eaten? Again, if assessing remotely, you may require the relative or carer to confirm this information.

As highlighted, considering the reason for the fall is vital, therefore understanding the intrinsic and extrinsic factors which may contribute to a fall or increase the risk of falls is essential. **Please note 'mechanical fall' is NOT an acceptable term**. Below are some of the more common factors; this list is not exhaustive. Chapter 7: Activities of Daily Living discusses the housing environment and the complex control it takes to walk, balance and stand in further detail.

Intrinsic Factors

Balance and Stability

Balance can be illustrated as being two functions. One distinguishes position in space and one returns the body to a balanced position (Darowski, 2008). Standing balance is known as 'static balance', whereas balance while moving is 'dynamic balance' which requires preparation, planning and judgement (Darowski, 2008). Nerves inform the brain of sensation, movement and position; however, these naturally deteriorate with age. Age-related decline in bodily sensations is thought to be an important risk factor for falls (Darowski, 2008).

Cardiac

Cardiac events may cause syncopal falls of which there are numerous examples. Cardiopulmonary and structural disease may cause cardiac events (MI, AFib, AS, aortic dissection) whereas a reduction in ventricular filling and stroke volume may lead to dysrhythmias (paroxysmal supraventricular tachycardia, atrioventricular conduction system blocks) (BMJ, 2022a).

Cognition

Cognition is essential to remaining upright, as it requires preparation, decision making and visuospatial awareness (Woodford, 2022). Additionally, attention, working memory, cognitive flexibility and inhibitory control are necessary for executive function which is vital for normal walking (Yogev-Seligmann et al., 2008). Therefore, those with executive dysfunction (long-standing, acute or increased) can experience a higher risk of falls (Yogev-Seligmann et al., 2008). They may have a baseline of unsteadiness, feel disoriented due to environmental changes, forget their functional limits or how to summon help (pendant alarms, 999 and others) (Woodford, 2022). Lack of concentration on balance can lead to falls, though this may be unavoidable due to small vessel disease affecting the brain (Darowski, 2008).

It is not always clear if patients have had an acute change in their cognition, therefore collateral information is vital. Family or carers may be able to advise if the patient is slower to process information, is drowsier than normal or is behaving unusually, all of which can point to possible delirium (Chapter 3: Frailty discusses delirium in more detail).

Dehydration

This may be rapid from significant fluid loss due to diarrhoea or vomiting, however many older people do not take on enough fluids in general meaning that any small stressor can cause them to become unwell and clinically dehydrated increasing their risk of falls. Assessment of dehydration in relation to thirst can be difficult in older people because as we age, due to decreased sensation, we may not feel as thirsty. This can be more significant in those with cognitive impairment, especially if they experience difficulty swallowing or drinking. Additionally, some patients with cognitive impairment will lose their sense of smell which also affects their sense of taste (Darowski, 2008). They may also stop their diuretics or reduce their fluid intake to prevent incontinence (Guy's and St Thomas's NHS Foundation Trust, 2023). Renal function is known to reduce from our forties (Aiello et al., 2017). In older adults this can be exacerbated due to multimorbidity and frailty further increasing the risk of dehydration (British Nutrition Foundation, 2023). This makes it challenging for older people to compensate for fluid and electrolyte imbalances (Woodford, 2022). Some medications may also exacerbate dehydration.

Fear of Falling

Not all people who have a fear of falling have had a fall (Preston et al., 2018) and a fear of falling is not just restricted to an individual, but may also be experienced by their family or carers (Darowski, 2008). A fear of falling may lead to reduced activities and therefore a potential reduction in muscle strength (Darowski, 2008) which can lead to an individual altering their gait, therefore possibly increasing the risk of falling producing a vicious cycle (Preston et al., 2018). Questionnaires have been utilised to help identify reasons for the fear, which have included loss of dignity and/or being alone and unable to get up (Darowski, 2008).

Feet

Good foot health is important for mobility and staying upright. Always consider the patient's foot health. Does someone cut their nails or do these hinder their balance and walking? Do they have neuropathy due to LTCs and therefore reduced sensory information?

Frailty

Individuals living with frailty are more predisposed to falling and the consequences of a first fall could be the start of living with frailty. See Chapter 3: Frailty for further explanation of frailty and further frailty syndromes.

Hypotension

If a person has fallen it is essential to assess their blood pressure and pulse, both lying and standing, to look for the causes and contributing factors. Patients with OH could present with syncopal or pre-syncopal symptoms. Older people are more susceptible to hypotension due to associated medications and comorbidities. OH is a progressive and constant fall in blood pressure from baseline that is symptomatic:

- Systolic: a drop of 20 mmHg or more or to less the 90 mmHg
- Diastolic: a drop of 10 mmHg or more.

It can be divided into neurogenic and non-neurogenic. Neurogenic OH includes conditions such as: Parkinson's disease, type 2 diabetes mellitus and small cell lung carcinoma (Rasanathan, 2020). Non-neurogenic OH usually occurs due to either venous pooling, hypovolaemia or cardiac failure (Figueroa et al., 2010). This can include conditions such as MI, AS, dehydration, adrenal insufficiency, fevers and many common medications for example, antihypertensive and diuretics amongst many (Rasanathan, 2020) (Chapter 6: Polypharmacy and Medicines Review has further information on medications).

Postural Orthostatic Tachycardia Syndrome

Postural orthostatic tachycardia syndrome (POTS) is the absence of OH, but with an increased heart rate of more than 30 bpm or an increase to more than 120 bpm within 10 minutes of active standing (NICE, 2023a). The aetiology is not fully understood and the severity of symptoms is variable. POTS is not limited to older people and can have an array of symptoms including inability to regulate temperature, palpitations and lethargy. It is usually diagnosed by specialists or consultants following referral.

Dizziness

Dizziness is vague and has many varied descriptions such as, wooziness, light-headedness, sensations of spinning or turning, unsteadiness, feeling like you are about to black out or are off balance (Newcastle Hospitals NHS Foundation Trust, 2020). However, Woodford (2022) simplifies this by dividing the varied descriptions into two categories: pre-syncope (a sensation of light-headedness) and vertigo (a feeling of movement, usually the room spinning). Pre-syncope is discussed throughout this chapter as many risk factors include pre-syncope symptoms, such as OH and cardiac causes. Vertigo can be triggered by irregular messages being sent from the inner ear on one side, leading to unbalanced data which the brain translates as rotating (Darowski, 2008). However, it can also be caused by lesions affecting the inner ear, vestibular nuclei in the brainstem or the vestibulocochlear nerve (Woodford, 2022). Diagnoses include benign paroxysmal positional vertigo (BPPV) (certain head movements cause vertigo), labyrinthitis (inner ear infection usually triggered by a virus), vestibular neuritis (inflammation of the vestibular nerve) and Ménière's disease (inner ear condition, which can involve tinnitus or hearing loss). Certain side effects of medication for migraines may be a causative factor (NHS, 2023b). It is important to be mindful of posterior circulation strokes which can present with acute, persistent, continuous dizziness or vertigo with nystagmus, new gait unsteadiness, nausea or vomiting and head motion intolerance (NICE, 2023c).

Illness

Acute illness or exacerbations of long-term diseases (of any origin) can weaken an individual, cause cardiac arrhythmias, blood pressure changes and/or abnormalities with their bloods, leading to a reduction in their functioning which can cause or increase confusion and/or pain. Always look for an underlying illness in a person who falls (Clegg et al., 2013). As previously mentioned, often older people do not present with classic symptoms, therefore an acute deterioration in their function or cognition can indicate an underlying medical cause for a fall. Many older people may present with a delirium as the first sign of illness. This may present as agitation, sleepiness, lack of engagement or a mixture of all of these. Delirium is discussed in more detail in the Chapter 3: Frailty. Blood tests, imaging and treatments are not always appropriate or even welcomed, but a robust face to face assessment needs to be considered including shared decision making with the patient, family and carers about what is important to them (Rockwood, 2021).

Incontinence

There is conflicting evidence regarding urinary incontinence being a causative factor of falls, however, a recent meta-analysis did establish urinary incontinence as a predictor for falls (Moon et al., 2021). Incontinence can affect mood and dignity. It can also lead to poor skin health and can affect quality of sleep (Woodford, 2022). A broader connection between incontinence and falls includes the issues incontinence can cause. For example hurrying to the toilet, nocturia when patients are drowsy or it is dark, urinary leakage on a hard floor causing a slip, medications to treat incontinence causing OH or reducing oral intake to prevent urinary frequency then becoming dehydrated. To prevent incidents outside, older people may reduce time away from their home, resulting in less activities, potentially leading to reduced body strength and isolation (Guy's and St Thomas's NHS Foundation Trust, 2023; Darowski, 2008). Acute urinary incontinence may be due to many issues (see Chapter 3: Frailty, for further information) the most significant of which being cauda equina syndrome. Therefore, it is important not to simply label incontinence as a urinary tract infection, but to exclude all significant pathology. Consider referral to a local bladder and bowel service.

Low Body Mass Index

This is often associated with malnutrition. Multimorbidity and chronic illnesses can influence a patient's capability or desire to eat, for example, they may experience reduced appetite and taste sensations, which can predispose individuals to malnutrition. Furthermore, ageing, frailty and physical challenges (holding cutlery, chewing, swallowing) can make an individual's ADLs and therefore mealtime habits difficult leading to reduced or poor nutrition (Holdaway and Nash, 2019). Consider referrals to dietetics or speech and language therapies.

Muscle Weakness

This is often accompanied by reduced function which may be gradual (general deterioration) or rapid in onset (during an acute episode of illness). Just think about how weak you feel when unwell with a virus or episode of vomiting. As we age, a reduction in the 'first responder' type of muscle fibres (Dawson-Hughes, 2017) and increased muscle adiposity are associated with deteriorating physical function (Lang et al., 2008). Prolonged time in bed can cause deconditioning for older adults (BGS, 2017). If you add deconditioning to a patient who has evidence of sarcopenia, then it demonstrates how a mild illness or injury could have significant impact on an older person's function. Furthermore, the individual may have pain, have had a debilitating event (stroke) or ongoing neurological disease-causing muscle weakness (see Chapter 7: Activities of Daily Living for further information).

Neurological

Certain conditions may be the cause of a fall, such as an acute stroke leading to an abrupt change in function, or it may be a long-term deterioration following a neurological event or disease. Strokes can cause loss of coordination, muscle weakness, impaired balance and/or judgement (Darowski, 2008). As mentioned, posterior circulation strokes can present with dizziness and can be difficult to identify. Symptoms of Parkinson's disease may cause falls due to motor and non-motor symptoms. Non-motor symptoms which increase the risk of falls include visual impairment, malnutrition, sarcopenia and cognitive impairment (Gupta and Shukla, 2021). Motor symptoms include rigidity, stiffness, bradykinesia and freezing (Parkinson's UK, 2023), which can all contribute to falls. Visual hallucinations have been evidenced as a cause of recurrent falls (Lima et al., 2022). Likewise, many dementias can present with similar risk factors, therefore a thorough exploration of a patient's medical history is essential.

Pain

This is often under reported by older people as they have learnt to live with, and adjust to, their daily aches and pains. Those with cognitive impairments may not be able to express their pain clearly, so look for subtle signs and utilise specific screening tools such as the Pain Assessment in Advanced Dementia Scale (PAINAID). Sufficient analgesia may reduce the risk of falling for active individuals and a tailored approach considering both pharmacological and non-pharmacological treatments should be considered (Montero-Odasso et al., 2022).

Vision

Approximately 75% of visual issues in older people are thought to be correctable through suitable glasses or surgery (Woodford, 2022). Visual problems can include reduced visual acuity, contrast sensitivity and depth perception amongst many conditions which affect how one visually interprets what is in front of them, for example, where the stairs finish (Darowski, 2008). Research has recognised contrast and depth perception, above visual acuity, as considerable risk factors for falls (Mehta et al., 2022).

Vitamin D Deficiencies

Though not a clear risk factor for falls, a Cochrane review concluded that 'vitamin D probably reduces the rate of falls, but probably makes little or no difference to the risk of falling' (Cameron et al., 2018). However, vitamin D works closely with calcium to protect bones. Vitamin D promotes bone health by facilitating the absorption of calcium from food. Together with calcium it helps protect against osteoporosis and aids effectiveness of the immune system and muscles (the National Institute of

Arthritis and Musculoskeletal and Skin Diseases, 2023), therefore demonstrating its usefulness in assisting with strong muscles which in turn assist with staying upright. A FRAX score is often completed to determine what intervention level is required, for example, treatment with medications or referral to a specialist bone clinic for a DEXA scan (National Osteoporosis Guidelines Group, 2021).

Walking and Gait

Approximately 60% of the over 80s, which increases to 82% in the over 85s, develop a gait disorder (Ronthal., 2019). Gait abnormalities can trigger following central (cerebrovascular or neurodegenerative) or peripheral (osteoarthritis) problems (Woodford, 2022). In addition, the inherent modification that older people take involves shorter strides and keeping both feet on the floor for longer (lifting the rear foot slower as the weight moves into the front foot) (Darowski, 2008). See Chapter 7: Activities of Daily Living for further information.

Extrinsic Factors

Lighting

Poor lighting (especially in long corridors without natural light or bathrooms without windows) may contribute to falls. Consider if the individual can change a ceiling light bulb or afford to replace one. Suggest night lights or motion detectors which illuminate areas during movements, especially bedrooms and bathrooms (Woodford, 2022).

Aids

An issue with varifocals is not seeing anything immediately in front of your feet so you can miss a pet, bag or step. Light changing lenses may not have adapted in time to allow clear vision of hazards. Walking sticks and walking frames can become hazards and increase falls if not used correctly or if they have fallen over.

Footwear

Loose, poorly fitting footwear, threadbare or reduced sole grip all contribute towards falls. If a shoe does not fit correctly, has opened toes or is inappropriate for the person and task, this can increase an individual's risk of falls.

Medications

Many medications are known to increase falls in older people and should be reviewed by a prescriber at every opportunity with an aim to deprescribe or reduce pertinent medications. There are several online lists which can help to identify the worst offenders. Always distinguish a patient's long-term medications as well as any new analgesics and consider that many medications are harsh on the ageing body (there is further information in Chapter 6: Polypharmacy and Medicines Review).

Alcohol and Non-Prescription Medications

Alcohol impairs processing of the brain and alcohol mixed with medications may exacerbate this issue (Darowski, 2008). Furthermore, alcohol, cannabis and non-prescription medications are increasing for the over 50s – a 23% rise in alcohol use and a 250% increase in cannabis in those over 65 years (Han et al., 2018).

Environment

What is the patient's environment like? Community and prehospital clinicians gain a wealth of information from observing patients within their own environment. Documenting a person's environment, clutter level and so on can be vital in assisting community teams to determine suitable equipment and potential challenges (see Chapter 7: Activities of Daily Living, for further information).

Complications of Falls

Some complications are also risk factors, such as dehydration and renal issues as previously discussed. The following are also complications regularly encountered.

Major Trauma

Falls from standing height are the most common cause of major trauma in older people (Trauma Audit and Research Network, 2017), with the most prevalent serious injuries being to the chest and head (Nickel et al., 2021). For more in-depth information refer to Chapter 9: Major Trauma.

Head Injuries

More than one million people attend EDs within England and Wales with a head injury. This is a significant cause of death and disability in those of less than 40 years old, however, older people (more than 65 years of age) are a growing ratio due to low-level falls (NICE, 2023b).

Ambulance services and health and care providers usually have their own local pathways to follow for head injuries and the following information is not to override policies and procedures but to increase knowledge of the older person's risk factors.

Ageing is associated with increasing risk factors for brain haemorrhages in relation to head injuries; these are summarised in Table 8.1.

Table 8.1 Increased risk of head injuries in older people.

Risk	Description
Cerebral atrophy	Increases the space between the arachnoid and dura mater leading to a vulnerability to rupture. This space may also result in delayed presentation of altered consciousness.
Hypertension	Hypertension leads to increased vessel wall tension therefore increased risk factor for aneurysm formation and blood vessel rupture.
Reduced cerebral autoregulation	Can cause diminished blood supply and hypoxic brain injury.
Cerebrovascular atherosclerosis	Increased risk of spontaneous intracerebral haemorrhage.
Ageing mitochondria	Can reduce the cerebral resilience to brain injury.

Source: based on Beedham et al., 2019.

The consequences of severe head injuries in older people can be significant and may lead to cerebral haemorrhage, of which a subdural haemorrhage is the most common occurring in more than 30% of severe head injuries (Abdi et al., 2023).

Older adults who have experienced a loss of consciousness or amnesia since the injury should be considered for a scan (NICE, 2023b; Rajesh et al., 2023). However, for some older patients, an urgent multi-specialty and multidisciplinary discussion involving family, carers and the patient may be necessary to determine the level of intervention required (Nickel et al., 2021). A simple question for the family or carers of a person living with severe frailty and/or cognitive impairment may be, what would they want? For further information on significant head injuries please see the Chapter 9: Major Trauma.

Fragility Fractures

Osteoporosis increases the risk of fragility fractures. From approximately 40 years of age, more bone cells are absorbed than are produced, meaning that bones lose density and become thinner (this process quickens for women post menopause) (Darowski, 2008). In addition, a direct relative with diagnosed osteoporosis or an individual's use of certain medications, such as steroids, means an increased risk of developing the disease (OHID, 2022). Hospital costs for hip fractures account for over £1 billion and approximately 1.8 million hospital bed days. This does not include the high cost of social care (OHID, 2022). It is important to remember osteoporotic fractures can occur with very little impact, even no impact. WHO suggest that a 'force from standing height' is enough to cause a fragility fracture (WHO, 2021). If a patient has a history of previous fragility fractures, they are prone to further fractures. Always consider a referral to a prescribing clinician who will be able to consider potential bone health investigations and treatments and/or their GP for a bone health review.

Long Lies

A long lie has been defined as 'anyone on the floor for over an hour and unable to get up' (JRCALC and AACE, 2022). Bloch (2012) states that remaining on the floor for a long period following a fall nearly doubles the possibility of death. A 2008 study examining falls in the over 90s reported that at least 30% were on the floor for 1 hour or more (Fleming and Brayne, 2008). Conditions associated with a long lie include pressure wounds, hypothermia, rhabdomyolysis, acute kidney injuries and dehydration (Bloch et al., 2008; JRCALC and AACE, 2022). Not all long lies are the same. Exploration is required regarding the patient's ability to reposition, sit or take fluids and a safeguarding referral should always be considered.

Pressure Wounds

Tissue damage may occur following either brief exposure to extreme pressure or continued exposure to minimal levels of pressure and can occur due to pressure, friction or moisture. It is essential causes are identified and patients are clinically assessed for appropriate treatments. Older adults are at a greater risk of pressure wounds because they can have a 20% thinner dermis (Haroun, 2003) and are more vulnerable to mild mechanical insult (International Review, 2010). Repositioning is key to removing the compression (Wilkinson et al., 2017). Always consider a safeguarding report if the patient has a pressure area.

Hypothermia

This can develop in some older adults who may be unable to identify temperature due to a loss of sensory receptors of the nerve endings in the dermis, epidermis and subcutaneous tissues as well as their environment, such as cold floors (concrete, tiles) or poorly or over heated residences (Nigam and Knight, 2017).

Rhabdomyolysis

Rhabdomyolysis may be the consequence of non-prescription or prescription medications, traumatic injury or medical events causing damage to the myocyte cells of skeletal muscle cells (BMJ, 2022b). Myocyte death triggers the release of myoglobin, urate, electrolytes and creatine kinase (CK) into the blood (Wallis, 2023): the consequences can include acute kidney injuries, electrolyte disturbances, acidaemia, disseminated intravascular coagulation and multi-organ failure (BMJ, 2022b).

Causes include traumatic (prolonged immobilisation or crush injuries) or non-traumatic extreme exertion (prolonged seizures), surgery (due to prolonged immobilisation or direct muscle ischaemia), drugs (statins, antipsychotics, illicit drugs), infections or inherited disorders (muscular dystrophy). Signs and symptoms may include dark urine (myoglobin stained, often described as 'tea' coloured, but is uncommon), muscle oedema and strains, muscle weakness, myalgias and malaise (BMJ, 2022b; Wallis, 2023).

Investigations include blood tests with the most specific being serum CK (a test used to detect damaged heart, skeletal or brain muscle (Medline Plus, 2023)). An increase of more than 5 times normal or more than 1,000 IU/L is a clinical classification rhabdomyolysis (BMJ, 2022b; Wallis, 2023), however, this can increase or reduce over several hours. Older people can be more prone to rhabdomyolysis following a fall due to being immobilised for long periods following an acute event (Marcus et al., 1992).

Clinical Investigations

These are dependent on your working environment, protocols, your resources, the cause of the fall and what the patient wants. JRCALC and AACE (2022) provide comprehensive guidance to assist those working within the ambulance sector. Baseline observations should be obtained to inform the NEWS2 (Royal College of Physicians, 2017) which will help to determine the acuity level of the patient. Always consider completing a 12-lead ECG (JRCALC and AACE, 2022).

Community teams and hospital investigations may also include routine blood tests. These usually include FBC, U&E, CRP which looks for sources of infection, anaemias, acute kidney injuries, electrolyte imbalance with potential added investigations to include liver function, bone and clotting studies. If the patient is acutely confused (see Chapter 3: Frailty, for more information on delirium) further blood tests may be requested, including glucose, magnesium, B12, folate and TFTs. Furthermore, a chest X-ray (usually within hospitals, but could be requested via the community teams) and a midstream urine sample (which should be sent for laboratory analysis, not a urine dip) may be requested to look for sources of infection. If the patient has experienced a potential 'long lie', a serum CK is also included. Often with older people many of their blood results are not 'typically normal', so it is important to assess their previous readings and look for acute abnormalities or slow deterioration which has now reduced to a level that may have contributed to a fall (such as low sodium).

Functional Assessments

The patient's function needs to be assessed following a fall (JRCALC and AACE, 2022). This is to determine if they are mobilising normally or if weight-bearing reveals any further injuries which may determine the appropriate outcome; for example, remain at home, occupational therapist, crisis response, admission to a frailty virtual ward, transport to the ED, same-day emergency care (SDEC) or frailty unit for further care. Chapter 7: Activities of Daily Living discusses functional assessment tools and considerations.

What Can We Do?

Firstly, it is essential that you utilise correct manual handling equipment and techniques to assist a patient from the floor (refer to your local guidelines) or consider how someone might assist the patient (for example, a family member following a remote assessment). As discussed, patients may experience a range of issues leading to a fall which could also cause them complications when being assisted from the floor. Those who have fallen are at risk of further falls (Health Direct, 2021) therefore, it is vital to identify patterns, such as time of day, dim lighting or vision issues (Woodford, 2022). In addition, review possible hazards (rugs, inappropriate aids) or potential changes required (bed lever, walking frame, vision review).

Your area of work and the patient's needs will determine who you are able to refer to. Safeguarding concerns must be addressed by considering and applying your local safeguarding policy (for further information, please refer to Chapter 12: Safeguarding). If within an ambulance service, a local falls referral pathway is often your first point of contact. If working within UCR or if you are part of a team that has been referred to, you need to consider who can help further. For example, you may need a referral to an occupational therapist to help determine easy changes such as the correct mobility equipment and aids, grab handles or banisters or the local authority for a falls activation alarm to prevent long lies. Always ensure a medications review has been instigated or requested. Most community teams have access to community pharmacists and many GP surgeries employ their own pharmacist.

Most hospitals have teams (usually called 'Frailty' or Older Persons Assessment and Liaison 'OPAL') that specialise in providing care for older people; these teams work across frailty units, ED, SDEC and acute medical admissions and usually comprise a geriatrician, ACPs, physiotherapists, occupational therapists and potentially a social worker. They utilise the CGA approach to assessing patients. Some frailty teams may be contactable from ambulance services and/or community teams directly to assist with shared decision-making. Furthermore, the development of virtual wards and direct access to SDEC departments can assist in reducing time in ED enabling the patient to remain at home with consultant-led care (NHS England and NHS Improvement, 2019; NHS, 2021b) (See Chapter 3: Frailty, for more information on frailty and CGAs).

CHAPTER 8 Falls

It is important to consider what matters to the patient and the level of frailty (Chapter 3: Frailty discusses screening for frailty) the individual is living with. This will assist in determining which referrals will be beneficial. Exercise and physical activity are advocated by NICE (2019). A Cochrane review which examined over 100 trials involving over 24,000 participants determined that exercise which focuses on muscle strength, balance and gait can help prevent falls in community-dwelling older people (Sherrington et al., 2020). Local authorities and some authority-run community centres offer falls prevention and/or strength and balance classes which patients can self-refer to, however to attend, individuals need to be mobile and able to exercise therefore the classes may not be accessible to those living with higher levels of frailty.

If you work within a community team, GP or outreach service you may consider referral to a falls clinic, usually run by a geriatrician (with a physiotherapist) to address both medical and functional causes of falls. If the patient has an LTC such as Parkinson's disease, dementia (undiagnosed or diagnosed), OH and so on, then referrals to specialist teams may benefit the patient.

In addition, literature which can assist the patient, families and carers may be the information they need to empower the individual to self-manage their risk factors.

Supporting families is essential, so always check that those who love and care for the patient are managing. There is a lot of community support available, but often people are overwhelmed and unsure where to look or who to trust. Most GP practices and communities have access to 'social prescribers' or 'care connectors' who will be able to assist patients and their families to access available services. Furthermore, they can also help the carer with contacts for the Carer's Trust or similar groups for support and assistance; for example, someone to sit with their loved one while they go shopping or even just sleep.

What Matters?

It is also vital to ensure that you understand 'what matters' to the individual and their support team. The NHS aims to provide personalised care empowering individuals to have options and control over how their care is delivered to support their needs (NHS, 2023a). Care needs to incorporate shared decision making combining the patient's and carer's points of view (Rockwood, 2021). Essential to shared decision making is ensuring information is not withheld but delivered in uncomplicated terms and involves both choice and support to make that choice (Rockwood, 2021).

Ethical Considerations

Beauchamp and Childress (2001) outlined the principles of biomedical ethics: beneficence, justice, non-maleficence and respecting patient autonomy. However, applying these values to older patients can be difficult due to varying levels of cognitive and physical impairment which cause reliance on family and carers (Nickel et al., 2021). An individual's capability to express their autonomous wishes can diminish with physical and cognitive decline. It is therefore critical to explore what is important to them and ensure suitable adaptations to assist with this (hearing, written) (Harley, n.d.; Nickel et al., 2021).

Conclusion

Nickel et al. (2021) suggests the following when exploring a person's autonomous decisions:

1. Do they know enough? (have they been sufficiently informed?)
2. Can they think enough? (is their cognitive ability or 'mental capacity' adequate?)
3. Are they free enough? (are they free from coercive influences?)

If you can answer 'yes' to all three questions then the individual's decision should be followed; if not, further exploration is required (Nickel et al., 2021).

Understanding 'what matters' and having a shared decision making approach to all care will assist with ethical issues as it allows a better understanding of the individual's wishes.

Conclusion

Falls are increasing alongside an ageing population; however, many falls can be prevented by addressing the predisposing factors alongside a multidisciplinary approach. Therefore it is essential that, as healthcare professionals, we utilise each contact to ask about falls.

Assessment of older people who have fallen needs to be comprehensive and make every effort to identify the type of fall (pre-syncopal, syncopal or non-syncopal) as well as identifying intrinsic and extrinsic factors. Awareness of an individual's risk factors will assist in identifying those at higher risk of frailty fractures.

It is necessary to refer individuals to specialist teams to enable a suitable assessment of an individual's falls risk (Montero-Odasso et al., 2022). For community-dwelling people, improving balance and building strength is an evidence-based intervention which can help reduce an individual's risk of falls. Therefore, informing the patient of available strength and exercise programmes will help to reduce further falls (Montero-Odasso et al., 2022; Sherrington et al., 2020). Always consider family, carers and loved ones in addition to the patient. Their stress and anxiety in relation to falls can be debilitating and lead to isolation for all.

Questions

1. Consider this chapter's content and apply what you have learnt to a recent patient. Was their fall pre-syncopal, syncopal or non-syncopal?
2. Thinking about this patient, did they have any frailty syndromes, polypharmacy or reduced function that contributed to their fall?
3. Think holistically, were there any extrinsic factors? How could you modify these to improve safety?

CHAPTER 8 Falls

Further Resources

- British Medical Journal (BMJ) Best Practice (2022). *Assessment of falls in the elderly*. Available at: https://bestpractice.bmj.com/topics/en-gb/880
- British Medical Journal (BMJ) Best Practice (2022). *Assessment of syncope*. Available at: https://bestpractice.bmj.com/topics/en-gb/248
- Montero-Odasso M et al. (2022). World guidelines for falls prevention and management for older adults: A global initiative. *Age and Ageing*, 51(9): 205.
- Sherrington C et al. (2019). Exercise for preventing falls in older people living in the community. *Cochrane Database of Sytematic Reviews*, 1: CD012424.

Resources for Your Patients and Their Families or Carers

- Age UK Advice line: 0800 678 1602. Lines are open 8am–7pm, 365 days a year. https://www.ageuk.org.uk/services/age-uk-advice-line/
- Age UK befriending services. Available at: https://www.ageuk.org.uk/services/befriending-services/
- Age UK. Available at: https://www.ageuk.org.uk/
- Dementia UK helpline: 0800 888 6678. Available at: https://www.dementiauk.org/contact-us-details/
- Lunch clubs – usually available on council and/or local Facebook group websites
- Silverline: A helpline for older people: 0800 4 70 80 90. Available at: https://www.thesilverline.org.uk/what-we-do/
- University of the Third Age (U3A): UK-wide movement of locally run interest groups that provide a wide range of opportunities to come together to learn for fun. Members explore new ideas, skills and activities together. Available at: https://www.u3a.org.uk/about

References

Abdi H, Hassani K, Shojaei S (2023). An investigation of cerebral bridging veins rupture due to head trauma. *Computer Methods in Biomechanics and Biomedical Engineering*, 26(7): 854–863.

Aiello E, Dueñas P and Musso CG (2017). Senescent Nephropathy: The New Renal Syndrome. *Healthcare*, 5(4), 81.

Beedham W, et al. (2019). Head injury in the elderly – an overview for the physician. *Clinical Medicine*, 19(2): 177–184.

Bloch F (2012). Critical falls: why remaining on the ground after a fall can be dangerous, whatever the fall. *Journal of American Geriatric Society*, 60(7): 1375–1376.

Bloch F, et al. (2008). Can metabolic abnormalities after a fall predict short term mortality in elderly patients? *European Journal of Epidemiology*, 24(7): 357–362.

British Geriatrics Society (BGS) (2017). Deconditioning awareness. Available at: https://www.bgs.org.uk/resources/deconditioning-awareness [accessed 27th September 2023].

References

British Medical Journal (2022a). Best practice: Assessment of syncope. Updated May 2022. Available at: https://bestpractice.bmj.com/topics/en-gb/248/pdf/248/Assessment%20of%20syncope.pdf[accessed 30th September 2023].

British Medical Journal (2022b). Best practice: Rhabdomyolysis. British Medical Journal Best Practice. BMJ Publishing Group Ltd. Available at: https://bestpractice.bmj.com/topics/en-gb/167/pdf/167/Rhabdomyolysis.pdf [accessed 30th September 2023].

British Nutrition Foundation (2023). Nutrition for Older People. Available at: https://www.nutrition.org.uk/nutrition-for/older-people/ [accessed 28th September 2024].

Cameron ID, et al. (2018). Interventions for preventing falls in older people in care facilities and hospitals. *Cochrane Database of Systematic Reviews*, 2018(9): CD005465.

Clegg A, et al. (2013). Frailty in elderly people. *The Lancet*, 381(9868): 752–762.

Clemson L, et al. (2023). Environmental interventions for preventing falls in older people living in the community. *Cochrane Database of Systematic Reviews*, 3(3): CD013258.

Darowski A (2008). *Falls*. Oxford: Oxford University Press.

Dawson-Hughes B (2017). Vitamin D and muscle function. *Journal of Steroid Biochemistry and Molecular Biology*, 173: 313–316.

Figueroa JJ, Basford JR, Low PA (2010). Preventing and treating orthostatic hypotension: as easy as A, B, C. *Cleveland Clinic Journal of Medicine*, 77(5): 298–306.

Fleming J, Brayne C (2008). Inability to get up after a falling, subsequent time on floor, and summoning help: prospective cohort study in people over 90. *British Medical Journal*, 337: a2227.

Ganz DA, Latham NK (2020). Prevention of falls in community-dwelling older adults. *The New England Journal of Medicine*, 382(8): 734–743.

Gupta S, Shukla S (2021). Non-motor symptoms in Parkinson's disease: opening new avenues in treatment. *Current Research in Behavioral Sciences* 2, Suppl 1: 14–20.

Guy's and St Thomas's NHS Foundation Trust (2023). Falls. Available at: https://www.guysandstthomas.nhs.uk/health-information/falls [accessed 28th September 2023].

Han BH, et al. (2018). Demographic trends of binge alcohol use and alcohol use disorders among older adults in the United States, 2005–2014. *Drug and Alcohol Dependence*, 170: 198–207.

Harley C (n.d.). General Medical Council video. Available at: https://www.gmc-uk.org/ethical-guidance/ethical-hub/older-adults#Older%20adults [accessed 28th May 2024].

Haroun MT (2003). Dry skin in the elderly. *Geriatrics and Aging*, 6(6): 41–44.

Health Direct (2021). Older people and falls. Available at: https://www.healthdirect.gov.au/falls#:~:text=A%20history%20of%20previous%20falls%20%E2%80%94%20If%20you,months%2C%20you%20are%20more%20likely%20to%20fall%20again [accessed 27th September 2023].

Holdaway A, Nash L (2019). Falls fact sheet. Integrating nutrition into falls pathways. Available at: https://www.malnutritionpathway.co.uk/falls.pdf [accessed 21st September 2023].

International Review (2010). Pressure ulcer prevention: pressure, shear, friction and microclimate in context. A consensus document. London: Wounds International, 2010. Available at: https://woundsinternational.com/consensus-documents/international-review-pressure-ulcer-prevention-pressure-shear-friction-and-microclimate-context/ [accessed 21st September 2023].

Joint Royal Colleges Ambulance Liaison Committee (JRCALC) and Association of Ambulance Chief Executives (AACE) (2022). *JRCALC Clinical Guidelines 2022*. Bridgwater: Class Professional Publishing.

Lang T, et al. (2008). Pelvic body composition measurements by quantitative computed tomography: association with recent hip fracture. *Bone*, 42(4): 798–805.

Lima. DP, et al. (2022). Falls in Parkinson's disease: the impact of disease progression, treatment, and motor complications. *Dementia and Neuropsychologica*, 16(2): 153–161.

CHAPTER 8 Falls

Marcus EL, Rudensky B, Sonnenblick M (1992). Occult elevation of CK as a manifestation of rhabdomyolysis in the elderly. *Journal of the American Geriatrics Society*, 40(5): 454–456.

MedlinePlus (2023). National Library of Medicine (US); creatine kinase. Available at: https://medlineplus.gov/lab-tests/creatine-kinase/ [accessed 28th May 2024].

Mehta J, et al. (2022). Visual risk factors for falls in older adults: a case-control study. *BMC Geriatrics*, 22(1): 134.

Montero-Odasso M, et al. (2022). Task Force on Global Guidelines for Falls in Older Adults. World guidelines for falls prevention and management for older adults: a global initiative. *Age and Ageing*, 51(9): afac205.

Moon S, et al. (2021). The impact of urinary incontinence on falls: a systematic review and meta-analysis. *PLoS ONE*, 16(5): e0251711.

National Institute for Health and Care Excellence (NICE) (2017). Falls in older people (NICE quality standard QS86). Available at: https://www.nice.org.uk/guidance/qs86/resources/falls-in-older-people-pdf-2098911933637 [accessed 27th September 2023].

National Institute for Health and Care Excellence (NICE) (2019). Surveillance of falls in older people: assessing risk and prevention (NICE guideline CG161). Available at: https://www.nice.org.uk/guidance/cg161/resources/2019-surveillance-of-falls-in-older-people-assessing-risk-and-prevention-nice-guideline-cg161-pdf-8792148103909 [accessed 2nd September 2023].

National Institute for Health and Care Excellence (NICE) (2023a). Blackouts and syncope. Available at: https://cks.nice.org.uk/topics/blackouts-syncope/ [accessed 30th September 2023].

National Institute for Health and Care Excellence (NICE) (2023b). Head injury: assessment and early management (NICE guideline NG232). Available at: https://www.nice.org.uk/guidance/ng232/resources/head-injury-assessment-and-early-management-pdf-66143892774085 [accessed 30th September 2023].

National Institute for Health and Care Excellence (NICE) (2023c). Stroke and TIA (summary). Available at: https://cks.nice.org.uk/topics/stroke-tia/#:~:text=Stroke%20and%20TIA%20generally%20present,non%2Dfocal%20or%20global%20deficits [accessed 12th April 2024].

National Institute of Arthritis and Musculoskeletal and Skin Diseases (2023). Calcium and vitamin D: important for bone health. Available at: https://www.niams.nih.gov/health-topics/calcium-and-vitamin-d-important-bone-health#:~:text=Vitamin%20D%20promotes%20bone%20health,our%20muscles%20and%20immune%20system [accessed 12 April 2024].

National Osteoporosis Guidelines Group, UK (2021). Clinical guideline for the prevention and treatment of osteoporosis. Available at: https://www.nogg.org.uk/full-guideline [accessed 20th September 2023].

Newcastle Hospitals NHS Foundation Trust (2020). Symptoms and treatment. Available at: https://www.newcastle-hospitals.nhs.uk/services/falls-and-syncope-service/symptoms-and-treatment/ [accessed 20th September 2023].

NHS (2021a). Falls. Available at: https://www.nhs.uk/conditions/falls/ [accessed 21st September 2023].

NHS (2021b). Guidance note. Frailty virtual ward (Hospital at Home for those living with frailty). Available at: https://www.england.nhs.uk/wp-content/uploads/2021/12/B1207-ii-guidance-note-frailty-virtual-ward.pdf [accessed 21st September 2023].

NHS (2023a). What is personalised care? Available at: https://www.england.nhs.uk/personalisedcare/what-is-personalised-care/ [accessed 27th September 2023].

NHS (2023b). Vertigo. Available at: https://www.nhs.uk/conditions/vertigo/ [accessed 21st September 2023].

NHS England and NHS Improvement (2019). Same-day acute frailty services. Available at: https://www.england.nhs.uk/wp-content/uploads/2021/02/SDEC_guide_frailty_May_2019_update.pdf [accessed 27th September 2023].

Nickel C, et al. (2021). *Silver book II: Geriatric syndromes*. Available at: https://www.bgs.org.uk/resources/silver-book-ii-geriatric-syndromes [accessed 27th September 2023].

References

Nigam Y, Knight J (2017). Anatomy and physiology of ageing 11: the skin. *Nursing Times*, 113(12): 51–55.

Office for Health Improvement and Disparities (OHID) (2022). Falls: applying all our health. Available at: https://www.gov.uk/government/publications/falls-applying-all-our-health/falls-applying-all-our-health [accessed 27th September 2023].

Parkinson's UK (2023). Motor symptoms of Parkinson's. Available at: https://www.parkinsons.org.uk/information-and-support/motor-symptoms-parkinsons [accessed 27th September 2023].

Preston J (2018). Fear of falling. The Hearing Aid Podcast. Episode 5.04. Available at: http://thehearingaidpodcasts.org.uk/5-04-fear-of-falling-3/ [accessed 10th September 2023].

Rajesh S, et al. (2023). Head injury: assessment and early management – summary of updated NICE guidance. Available at: https://www.bmj.com/content/bmj/381/bmj.p1130.full.pdf [accessed 21st September 2023].

Rasanathan D (2020). Postural hypotension in older adults. Geeky Medics. Available at: https://geekymedics.com/postural-hypotension-in-older-adults/ [accessed 28th September 2023].

Rockwood K (2021). *Silver Book II: Frailty*. Available at: https://www.bgs.org.uk/resources/silver-book-ii-frailty [accessed 28th September 2023].

Ronthal M (2019). Gait disorders and falls in the elderly. *Medical Clinics*, 103(2): 203–213.

Royal College of Physicians (2017). National Early Warning Score (NEWS) 2: Standardising the assessment of acute-illness severity in the NHS. Available at: https://www.rcplondon.ac.uk/projects/outputs/national-early-warning-score-news-2 [accessed 2nd September 2023].

Sherrington C, et al. (2020). Exercise for preventing falls in older people living in the community: an abridged Cochrane systematic review. *The British Journal of Sports Medicine*, 54(15): 885–891.

Trauma Audit and Research Network (2017). Major trauma in older people. Available at: https://aace.org.uk/wp-content/uploads/2017/04/Major-Trauma-in-Older-People-2017.pdf [accessed 28th September 2023].

Wallis J (2023). Rhabdomyolysis. Available at: https://geekymedics.com/rhabdomyolysis/ [accessed 28th September 2023].

Whitledge JD, et al. (2023). Presyncope. NCBI Bookshelf. A service of the National Library of Medicine, National Institutes of Health. StatPearls. Available at: https://www.ncbi.nlm.nih.gov/books/NBK459383/?report=printable [accessed 28th September 2023].

Wilkinson I, et al. (2017). Preventing pressure ulcers. Series 3 Episode 3. The Hearing Aid Podcasts. Available at: http://thehearingaidpodcasts.org.uk/wp-content/uploads/2017/03/shownotes-episode-3.3-Pressure-ulcers-3.pdf [accessed 10th September 2023].

Woodford HJ (2022). *Essential Geriatrics* (4th edition). Oxon: CRC Press.

World Health Organization (WHO) (2021). Falls. Available at: https://www.who.int/news-room/fact-sheets/detail/falls [accessed 2nd September 2023].

Yogev-Seligmann G, Hausdorff JM, Giladi N (2008). The role of executive function and attention in gait. *Movement Disorders*, 23(3): 329–342.

Zazzara MB, et al. (2021). Probable delirium is a presenting symptom of COVID-19 in frail, older adults: a cohort study of 322 hospitalised and 535 community-based older adults. *Age and Ageing*, 50(1): 40–48.

Chapter 9

Major Trauma

Duncan Robertson

Learning Points

By the end of this chapter, you will:

- Recognise the common mechanism of injury causing major trauma for older people
- Comprehend how trauma in older people presents compared to younger populations
- Appreciate how decisions on scene can affect the patient pathway
- Grasp how clinically complex older people are and how these complexities need to be considered as part of the assessment in major trauma
- Understand how trauma tools can under-triage older people.

Case Study

Background: It is midday on a Saturday in autumn. You are a solo paramedic cycle responder called to a city-centre pedestrianised area for male older adult who has been in a collision with an e-scooter.

When you arrive, you find a man called Tom on the floor with a blanket over him. He is 82 years old. You find out that he was walking, with the aid of a stick, in the shopping precinct having been for a hearing test, when a young adult on an e-scooter collided with him and knocked him sideways to the floor. The rider is uninjured, on scene and very apologetic, saying he shouted before impact, but it was too late.

Presenting Complaint: On initial examination Tom is conscious and alert and breathing normally but wincing in pain. He is well perfused and a nice pink colour. Despite the noise around you, he can hear you and communicating with him does not require a lot of adaptation to ensure you both understand each other. He does not appear to be confused.

CHAPTER 9   Major Trauma

He has a skin tear to the bridge of his nose and above his left eye is a laceration and a developing swelling. He holds broken spectacles in one hand and there are grazes to his palm from where he tried to break his fall. A bystander says that he seemed to be knocked out but came round very quickly.

He can move all four limbs. He has hit his head on the hard floor but managed to put his hands out to break some of the impact. He is mainly complaining of left sided rib pain as he landed on that side on top of his elbow, which dug in.

There is no pain or tenderness to his cervical spine, which has a full range of movement and his back is also pain free. He has no evidence of limb fractures or pain to his pelvis. There is no bruising to his chest, but he is tender on palpation to his left ribcage just below the level of the xiphisternum across three lower ribs.

As you assess him, he can speak in full sentences. His vision is unaffected, he is not pale, not sweaty and not short of breath. His pupils are equal and reactive to light and he does not complain of any nausea. He struggles to take a full inhalation which he says is due to the pain in his ribs, but on auscultation you hear good air entry to all lung fields and see equal chest movement.

Assessment

Pulse: 98 bpm and regular

Oxygen Saturations: 95%

Respiratory Rate: 22 regular breaths per minute

Blood Pressure: 105/86 mmHg

Temperature: 37.0°C

Pain Score: 7/10 pre-analgesia

Frailty score: CFS score 3

Previous Medical History: AFib, hypertension

Drug History: Amlodipine (5 mg once daily), rivaroxaban (20 mg once daily), atenolol (50 mg once daily), atorvastatin (20 mg once daily)

You administer analgesia to help with the rib pain: this seems to have an effect and Tom can breathe easier as a result and his oxygen saturations begin to climb to 98%.

Your working impression is that Tom has experienced a trauma. It is likely that he has rib fractures of an unknown number but can move some air and there is no evidence of a pneumothorax. You are worried that he has sustained a head injury, but there are no physiological changes to indicate a traumatic brain injury or a bleed.

Introduction

> Control message to say that an ambulance has been dispatched and while you await their arrival, you call the regional trauma desk as Tom does not immediately trigger bypass to enable access to the major trauma centre (MTC) – however, the clinician on the desk recommends a pre-alert to the MTC as Tom has sustained a head injury, has lost consciousness and is on a DOAC, with an increased risk of either a traumatic brain injury or an intracranial bleed. The chest injury will require treatment to ensure that Tom is able to clear secretions as he is at increased risk of pneumonia and respiratory failure. Tom is also taking a beta-blocker which may affect how his pulse rate is able to adjust to the physiological demands of his injuries. It is likely that Tom has sustained a major trauma. Upon arrival at the MTC, a scan indicates a ruptured spleen which required surgery.

Introduction

The nature of trauma care has changed considerably over the last four decades. From the baseline of a historical system designed to 'scoop and run' patients with traumatic injuries to the nearest ED, there now exist sophisticated systems designed to deliver specialist trauma care 24 hours a day, 7 days a week.

What is increasingly apparent in the UK is that the patterns of major trauma experienced by the population are changing. Effective data collection coordinated by the Trauma Audit and Research Network (TARN) has provided a more detailed understanding of the patterns and presentations of trauma and major trauma in particular. The 2017 report into trauma in older adults demonstrates clearly that our traditional thinking, that major trauma is a disease of the young and caused by high kinetic energy transfer through standard mechanisms of injury (such as RTCs, falls from height and so on), needs to be challenged. The evidence now firmly illustrates that the most prevalent group within the major trauma registry are adults over the age of 65 with the most prevalent mechanism of injury being a fall from standing, with head injuries being the most common injury type.

It is therefore important that we include this chapter on major trauma in older people. We will cover the understanding of trauma from the data and the need to follow a systematic approach to assess the patient. The assessment will follow some of the principles of the Advanced Trauma Life Support (ATLS) approach, but also incorporate elements from the Heartlands Elderly Care Trauma & Ongoing Recovery Programme (HECTOR) manual (Raven, 2019) which is an approach to trauma care designed specifically for clinicians providing care for older people. For community-based clinicians, having this awareness of what is major trauma will help with clinical decision making on scene and an understanding of the complexity that exists with older patients. The chapter is designed to be introductory and readers with interest in this area are recommended to download the HECTOR manual, attend a course and follow up with the podcasts listed in the resources at the end of the chapter.

CHAPTER 9 Major Trauma

What is Major Trauma and How Do We Identify It?

Major trauma is defined as an injury or combination of injuries that are life-threatening and could be life changing because it may result in long-term disability (NICE, 2016a). In the UK, there is a bimodal age distribution of major trauma, with the first peak in the under 20 group and a second in the over 65 group. For the purposes of data collection and service design, major trauma is identified with the retrospective application of the Injury Severity Score (ISS). For an injury or injuries to be considered major trauma, the score must be greater than 15.

As the ISS cannot be readily calculated at the scene of injury, ambulance services and trauma networks use agreed trauma triage tools, designed to identify the patients who will benefit the most from a decision to bypass the nearest facility to transfer directly to the major trauma centre (MTC). These tools use a mixture of metrics to aid decisions, including a measurement of vital signs following the <C>ACBDE (catastrophic haemorrhage, airway, c-spine, breathing, disability, expose and examine) approach, the anatomy of the injury and then the mechanism of injury.

However, despite these tools, we know there are practice gaps as more older people have their care provided in trauma units. Caroline Criado Perez in her 2019 book *Invisible Women* makes the case that the developments of roads and particularly car safety are based on data derived from male patterns of injury and crash test data that are biased towards male physiology and anatomy. This principle is recognised in trauma care. The tools developed to identify patients suitable for major trauma and bypass to MTCs were designed to capture trauma for a standard or normal physiology, that of a younger adult on no medications, or without significant disease burden. As such, the tools do not consider complex comorbidities or polypharmacy. Subsequent alterations to the major trauma tools include the addition of 'silver trauma' screening, but this too may lack the sensitivity and specificity required to capture a large group of patients who experience major trauma differently to younger, fitter, less frail and more robust counterparts.

As a result, older adults are at greater risk of under-triage and may miss out on the early interventions in definitive care that will lead to a greater chance of a full rehabilitation and return to normal baseline functionality. In other chapters we have explored how the changes in anatomy and physiology, living with complex comorbidities, the gradual loss of functional reserves, polypharmacy and frailty can have an impact on how people age. The fact that none of this is necessarily linear, nor directly related to age, means that predicting the severity of injury based on factors more readily applied to younger populations can be problematic. There exists a real risk of not identifying when trauma in older adults is in fact major trauma. Therefore, it is recognised by system experts that trauma is not the same in older populations compared with younger populations.

Age Differences

The application of biological age to this population does not necessarily reflect the reality of the lived experience. In deprived areas, the threshold of ageing might well be significantly lower than in less deprived areas. Understanding ageing processes and theories of frailty will enable the responder to have a more nuanced appreciation of clinical risk of injury and the potential for major trauma than the assumption that older age equals worse outcome. From the 2017 TARN data, older adults have a similar ISS in major trauma and are equally likely to recover to their baseline in comparison with younger cohorts.

However, with age come physiological changes that mean older people, particularly if living with frailty, dementia or other LTCs, are more at risk of major trauma from comparatively reduced kinetic forces, or mechanisms of injury, than younger cohorts. As Alqarni et al. (2023) outline, frailty has a better value in predicting adverse outcomes from major trauma than age alone, so clinicians likely to encounter major trauma should be familiar with the changes associated with ageing outlined in other chapters in this book.

Patterns in the Data

The 2017 TARN report on Major Trauma in Older People offers a clear insight into how our perceptions of the spread of major trauma across our population should be reconsidered.

Falls of less than 2 metres represent the mechanism for less than 20% of people aged 16–59. Between 60 and 69 years of age this rises to just over 40% and with each age band increases. In the 90+ category it represents over 80% of the recorded mechanisms. By contrast the road traffic collision (RTC) proportion drops from just over 40% of 16–59-year-olds to less than 10% of the 90+ group. These patterns suggest a difference in behaviour, but also link to the volume of falls-related activity that is described in more detail in Chapter 8: Falls. What else is striking from the report is that the location of major trauma is predominantly outdoors for 16–59-year-olds, but this changes to indoors from the age of 70 onwards and increases with age. Again, it is suggestive of the fact that older people may remain in the home and not seek to engage in risky activities, but in doing so, might be more susceptible to deconditioning, leading to loss of coordination and balance and hence more likely to fall from standing in the home environment.

As well as this understanding, analysis of the data indicates that many of these cases are not being seen in the MTCs, but the trauma units (Dixon et al., 2022). This has implications for the delivery of effective trauma care. The reasons behind this are that MTCs, when activated, will bring a team approach, led by a consultant, aimed at assessing the patient with a view towards initiating early interventions including imaging and scans to detect injury more accurately and, if required, immediate referral to surgery for lifesaving treatment. The trauma units, on the other hand, do not necessarily have the same approach and patients are initially assessed by more junior doctors (albeit experienced physicians) who then have to navigate the patient, and the involvement of a consultant may come at a much later stage of the care pathway. As such, the data indicate that older adults who enter a trauma unit wait longer to be assessed, wait longer for scans and wait longer for definitive treatment; for example, neurosurgery (TARN, 2017). Therefore, decisions made on scene can significantly affect the patient pathway and the timeliness of care delivery.

CHAPTER 9 Major Trauma

However, the reasons for this are complex and are traceable to the tools used to identify major trauma. These were designed on the effects that significant mechanisms of injury have on normal adult physiology. We have seen in other chapters of this book that the principles of normal physiology cannot be readily applied to a population who are more complex, have more diagnosed comorbidities, take more medications and have different physiologies including lower bone density and reduced skin elasticity and muscle mass. Later in the chapter we will see how other anatomical changes associated with old age can further complicate the picture and reduce the predictive probability that normal trauma tools will capture major trauma in our patient group.

Dixon et al. (2022) highlight the variation in numbers and patient characteristics within the UK major trauma system, but also demonstrate that older adults dominate UK major trauma and that there is a need to address variations and shortfalls in care. Prior to the TARN report of 2017, Kehoe et al. (2015) described the change in major trauma aetiology, from a disease of young men caused by high energy transfer mechanisms to a greater proportion of older adults, with the most common mechanism being low falls. Despite this knowledge, major trauma systems have been slow to adapt to the common presentations and the tools used to identify or exclude major trauma are still based on presentations in younger and more robust populations. Adaptations to trauma tools have included recommendations for older adults, however, their prognostic accuracy can be challenged with the higher volume of patients with major trauma being cared for in the trauma units rather than MTCs (Dixon, 2019).

What We Understand Now About Trauma

Providing trauma care for older adults is not as straightforward as following the ATLS algorithm without some critical thought. It requires a great degree of detective work to consider the full effects of the obvious injury and the consequences of missing a less obvious injury. The level of attention to detail is always important for clinicians in the community, however for this group of patients it is arguably more so, not only to consider the possibilities of injuries that would be expected given a particular mechanism of injury, but also injuries that may remain hidden due to the factors described in other chapters in the book.

Older adults are susceptible to the sequalae of traumatic events and it is important to recognise that trauma may not always be the physical, but also encompasses the emotional response. In Chapter 8: Falls, we can see that the psychological impact of a fall is often harder to deal with for the individual compared to the physical injuries sustained. This leads to a fear of leaving the home environment and a fear of being hospitalised. When speaking to an older person who has sustained an injury, they may be reluctant to attend hospital and so effective communication and a thorough understanding of the risks involved in order to make a truly informed decision is important to consider as well as checking that the injured person has the capacity to understand the information being provided.

Approaches to Trauma Assessment

ATLS and the HECTOR manual describe differing approaches to trauma care. ATLS is a sequential, structured approach to trauma care and one that focuses on technical skills to enable the rapid treatment of given injuries. The philosophy of the HECTOR approach is to apply critical reasoning to trauma in this group to allow for the differences in presentation that may affect how trauma is treated. As such, their approach is to 'treat a patient with injuries and not the injuries on a patient' (Raven, 2019).

The following section briefly covers the structured assessment of major trauma through the lens of the older adult. It does not cover the details of specific in-hospital tests and interventions, nor does it cover those deployed by critical care specialists who operate outside the hospital but is designed for the community-based clinician to be able to begin to understand the complexity within a <C>ACBCDE approach to trauma care.

It is important to document all injuries when undertaking a secondary survey and identify any non-accidental injury. Actively look for patterns of bruising inconsistent with the described mechanism of injury, or bruises or injuries of varying ages. If you suspect non-accidental injury, or injuries sustained by abuse, that person should have their safeguarding concerns reported to appropriate professionals for further support. This is outlined in more detail in Chapter 12: Safeguarding.

Catastrophic Haemorrhage

Consider the quantity of blood thinning medications that the older adult population are prescribed to prevent cardiovascular and neurovascular insult and it is easy to see how there is an increase in the risk of a catastrophic haemorrhage for older adults. Epistaxis and ruptured varicose veins can, if uncontrolled for a period, lead to significant blood loss, especially if the affected person is not able to control the bleeding themselves with the application of direct pressure. While it can be easy for a younger person to apply pressure, for a person with reduced strength, coordination, vision or living with mild cognitive impairment, a seemingly innocuous injury could present as life-threatening if help is not available immediately. Given that older adults are less likely to be able to compensate for large volumes of blood loss and may mask physiological signs of shock, such bleeds, without appropriate control, can lead to preventable deterioration.

Airway and Cervical Spine

When managing the airway of an older adult, special considerations include the presence of arthritis at the temporo-mandibular joint that may affect mouth opening. This will affect the ability to examine the airway for foreign bodies, positioning for effective suctioning and the use of adjuncts including the use of advanced airways. In addition, arthritic changes to the cervical spine will affect the ability to position the airway, including simple manoeuvres such as the head tilt and chin-lift. Loss of tone to facial and neck structures can also lead to airway compromise from the tongue.

CHAPTER 9 Major Trauma

Dentures can be a help in managing to position and secure an airway, unless they are broken or poorly fitting, in which case they can lead to further causes of airway obstruction. Teeth may be missing and those present held in reduced alveolar bone of the upper and lower jaw, with little force being required to dislodge them and again, causing a potential obstruction.

Changes to the bone structure of the neck may mean the person is at increased risk of a neck injury following a relatively innocuous mechanism of injury; be particularly cautious of the fractured odontoid peg. Older people who fall and are unable to use their hands to absorb the impact may be at risk of hyperextension injuries, leading to central cord syndrome. If a neck injury is suspected, immobilisation can be a challenge. However, guidelines indicate that best achievable position is preferred rather than attempting full in-line immobilisation with collar, blocks and scoop. It might be pragmatic to retain the patient's best position, being mindful of the affected anatomy where a patient may have marked kyphosis or scoliosis. In these cases, the use of rolled blankets or a vacuum mattress can provide the necessary support. Rigid collars can cause problems if incorrectly measured or poorly applied, including the risk of raising intracranial pressure or, following prolonged application, pressure injuries to skin and soft tissues. Be sensitive to the needs of the patient and exercise caution when immobilising to prevent further pain, further discomfort or further injury. If a patient is not able to tolerate immobilisation due to anxiety, agitation or confusion, adopt the best available positioning, aiming to reduce additional movement in a compassionate way.

Breathing

Common respiratory disease and illnesses can affect breathing in older adults and therefore their ability to effectively exchange gases to maintain homeostasis. In addition, ageing can affect the lung volume available for gaseous exchange. This reduction in respiratory reserve, means older adults are not able to compensate as well as younger people and may require supplemental oxygen therapy sooner. Remember that older adults with COPD are at risk of type 2 respiratory failure with the administration of excessive oxygen, so aim for target saturations in this group should oxygen be required, and do not immediately administer high-flow oxygen therapy.

Changes to bone density can make individuals more at risk of rib fractures, which can affect the rate and depth of inspiration. Increased skeletal rigidity leads to reduced chest wall compliance which leaves the older individual more at risk of injury as forces are not so easily dissipated across the whole chest wall. This leads to increased risk of focussed chest injury including contusions and haemorrhage. Rib fractures are associated with an increased risk of complications and death in older patients. We can see this in the case study above, where a falling force led to Tom's elbow digging into his chest wall and fracturing several ribs. If the extent of the rib fractures is such that Tom cannot effectively cough, he is at greater risk of developing pneumonia and respiratory failure as a result. This can increase his risk of mortality.

An older breathless patient who has had a chest trauma should be assessed for pneumothorax or haemothorax (or the presence of both – a pneumo-haemothorax).

This may not be readily apparent while on scene, so maintaining a high index of suspicion is important.

Circulation

Changes associated with normal ageing can lead to reduced cardiac output. For example, the myocardium effectively stiffens and the person is less able to respond to stressors by raising their heart rate or stroke volume leading to patients being unable to effectively compensate for excessive blood loss. As outlined in the HECTOR manual, the stiffening of blood vessels, desensitisation of baroreceptors and impaired autonomic function can further reduce the cardiac reserve and prevent effective compensation for blood loss.

Medications such as beta-blockers can reduce pulse rates to the extent that there is masking of the true symptoms. This will significantly affect the usefulness of physiological monitoring tools, such as a trauma tool or the NEWS2. This leads to the under-triage of older adults who are sick and actively compensating following a significant injury as their vital signs may appear in normal ranges. In addition, comorbidities or long-term diseases may lead to older adults living with raised blood pressure and a reading in trauma that may appear normotensive could in fact represent hypotension in the older adult.

Adjusted major trauma screening tools that accommodate older people indicate that a systolic blood pressure of under 110 mmHg should be considered as hypotension, compared to below 90 mmHg for younger adults. As a result, clinical decisions should be based on trends of observations rather than one-off readings and be assessed in the context of the patient's previous medical history.

Disability

Unrecognised head injuries in older adults are a real risk. As we age, the brain will atrophy, with a commensurate build-up of cerebrospinal fluid. This has protective properties in that it helps prevent contusions, however there is an increase in the risk of unrecognised bleeds (intracranial and subdural haemorrhage). These bleeds often result from rapid deceleration forces including falls from standing. This is because the atrophied brain still has the same vasculature, which earlier in life would have been intimately connected to the brain, but due to the shrinkage is under more tension as it is effectively suspended. Unlike a younger adult, who will show typical neurological signs early with a bleed (unequal pupils, reduced level of consciousness), the fact that there is increased space for the bleed to develop into without compromising the structure of the brain until later means there is a delay in such symptoms establishing themselves in the older adult cohort. The risk of bleeding is increased in those older adults who are prescribed anticoagulants or antiplatelets.

Kehoe et al. (2016), through their analysis of TARN data, demonstrate that GCS score is higher in older patients presenting with equivalent intracranial injury compared with younger age groups. This means that trauma tools that rely on GCS score as a parameter will under-perform for older adults and potentially put them at greater risk. Levels of consciousness can also be affected by LTCs such as dementia, but also due to the presence of delirium. Delirium can be present in trauma. The PINCHES

CHAPTER 9 Major Trauma

ME mnemonic outlining the potential causes of delirium includes Pain first. Effective treatment of pain can reduce the likelihood of developing delirium further down the patient pathway (see also analgesia, below).

Nicholson et al. (2022) highlight the difficulties experienced by paramedics when considering conveyance decisions for older adults with a minor head injury. Their study highlighted the perceived ambiguity of guidelines seemingly not written for a patient population with higher levels of frailty and what the consequences would be for not adhering to guidelines, balanced by the need for patient-centred decision making. 'Important factors included: the patient's social situation; guidelines; clinical support availability; the history and presentation of the patient [as well as] risk.' While some patients are candidates for surgery, others may require conservative treatment, however, these decisions are usually made following imaging, Therefore, there is the requirement in best practice guidelines to consider transfer to secondary care.

As well as cervical spine injuries, the spinal column is subject to bony changes in later life, with exacerbations of kyphosis and scoliosis, meaning that in-line immobilisation may not be possible. JRCALC guidelines indicate that a best attempt approach to immobilisation be used, with the aim to keep the patient still and maintaining their natural posture (JRCALC and AACE, 2022). While osteoporosis and osteoarthritis increase the risk of spinal fractures, these changes can also lead to a reduction in the spinal canal with an increase in the risk of injury to the spinal cord.

Long-standing conditions can lead to neurological changes; for example, neuropathy, which can mask the extent of how injuries are experienced and reduce the experience of pain. This can lead to patients seemingly underplaying their injuries or not realising the severity.

Exposure

With any injury, it is important to assess the skin of the patient. Due to age-related changes a reduction in collagen leads to skin being thinner and more prone to damage, either as a direct result of the traumatic incident or indirectly as a result of pressure damage. This damage is caused by lying on a hard surface for too long or by incorrect positioning and assessment of positioning by responders. Not only that, but skin changes also mean older adults are at increased risk of hypothermia (particularly if they need to be undressed to examine injuries) and infections. When examining a patient at the scene of an injury, be mindful of their dignity if you need to examine for a secondary survey but be aware of the onset of hypothermia if they have been outside for a long time and cover undressed areas with blankets while examining them to prevent further heat loss.

Burns

Older people are at greater risk of burn injuries compared to the wider population from multiple factors. While safety in terms of domestic heating and kitchen appliances are much improved, older people may not use up-to-date appliances and have a different perception of risk based on lived experience and habits. As a result, and due to reduced mobility, reduced reactions, loss of hearing and reduced vision, the risk of sustaining thermal injuries are increased while cooking or using heating. In addition, peripheral neuropathies may reduce the ability of the individual to know when they are at greatest risk of burns, and degrees of developing (or established) cognitive impairment may limit the ability to deal with risks as they emerge.

Older adults have a higher mortality than younger people with burn injuries which is linked to the total body surface area affected. The HECTOR manual outlines the predictors of mortality as including severity and number of comorbid illnesses, pre-existing malnutrition, post burn complications and increasing age. For a patient with a burn injury, a structured assessment should be followed, with the safety of the responder and the patient in mind. Stop the burning process and cool the burn, being mindful of hypothermia in patients who may not be able to effectively thermoregulate. Cover the burns with a cling film dressing and assess the airway for burns or potential inhalation injury; assess breathing and be aware of circumferential burns of the chest; administer analgesia following local protocols, and assess the total body surface area of the burn (there are applications and diagrams to help this stage of the process) and the depth of the burn injuries. For older adults, gaining a history is important in terms of how the injury was sustained and also a medical history, especially for diabetes and peripheral vascular disease.

Pelvis and Hip Injuries

Fractured neck of femur (NOF) is a common injury, with over 70,000 occurring each year in the UK (NICE, 2016b). Typically presenting with the affected limb being shortened and externally rotated, there are other injuries that can also occur in this area that may not be obvious until imaging has taken place. These include pubic rami fractures as well as fractures to the proximal femoral midshaft, which may mimic a NOF. These injuries have a high level of morbidity, however with rapid treatment pathways, patients can return to baseline following surgery and rehabilitation.

With these injuries, analgesia is important to administer as soon as possible. While the patient is likely to be holding themselves in a position where they can cope with the pain, they will need analgesia for any manual handling that will be required to get them from the scene into an ambulance, and then the subsequent transfers from ambulance to ED trolley and then for imaging. Therefore, non-pharmacological techniques used to support initial assessment must then be supplemented by appropriate use of analgesics based on local availability and scope of practice. Commencing a rapid acting inhalant will work effectively for older adults, but be mindful that for the more frail or confused patients they may not be able to follow instructions, either due to confusion or being unable to physically create the vacuum for delivery, particularly for nitrous oxide (Entonox).

Abdominal Injuries

Abdominal structures are subject to loss of protective mechanisms such as decreased abdominal wall muscle mass, reduction in bone density of the spine, lower ribs and pelvis, and therefore this area should have a high index of suspicion if affected by trauma, indicated by mechanism of injury or evidence of direct injury (wounds or bruising present). The abdomen has a large capacity and can mask blood loss. Physical examination may not be enough and patients with a suspected abdominal injury should be assessed in a facility with scanning options (ultrasound or CT-scan). Consider our older adult who is on a DOAC, a blood thinning medication. In our case study, the focal injury to Tom's ribs also overlays the spleen, meaning he was at increased risk of a splenic injury – not easy to identify on scene, but to consider as part of the examination.

Pain Management

Inadequate administration of analgesia is inhumane. Effective analgesia will reduce pain and anxiety in the patient and may also reduce the likelihood of a later delirium. Each service should select analgesia that best suits their practitioners, scope of practice and availability of medications. Routes of administration should be varied to enable the clinician to adopt a 'step-up' approach to the analgesic ladder. In addition, where permitted, nerve blocks may provide better and focussed relief of symptoms of isolated injuries compared to those analgesics which have more systemic effects. For the latter group of medications, when considering which to administer, the pharmacodynamics and pharmacokinetics of absorption, distribution, metabolism and excretion should be key considerations (see Chapter 6: Polypharmacy and Medicines Review). Trauma induces stress on the systems and will generate a systemic response. As such, gut motility is likely to be reduced, which will reduce the absorption of oral medications. In addition, there is a risk that, by asking the older person with trauma to take an oral medication, they could vomit, or also be at risk of airway complications should they require immediate surgery on arrival at the MTC. Therefore, with Tom, despite the indication of a head injury and chest injury, he might benefit more from the considered administration of an intravenous or inhaled analgesia over oral medications. Always use the most appropriate pain assessment tool for the patient based on local guidance.

Conclusion

Major trauma screening tools are not sufficiently sensitive to the needs of older adults, based as they are on the 'normal' physiological parameters of younger adults. Therefore, as we have seen through this chapter, the need for thoroughness is particularly important for our group of interest.

Treat the patient with injuries, rather than injuries on the patient and, as recommended in the HECTOR manual, be the clinician with a basic understanding of managing acute medical illness as this will positively help assessment. As we have seen, trauma is not only caused by acute medical illness, but the sequelae of trauma will also be affected by physiological changes associated with ageing and comorbidities. For the treatment of major trauma in older people, we need to have a high index of suspicion that a low mechanism of injury will have a bigger effect on the older adult; as such we need to be flexible in our approaches to provide more individualised care. As much as a structured ATLS approach will help us, it can also limit us and lead to the older patient receiving delayed care through the application of the wrong trauma pathway. Be a detective, be thorough and be questioning of the findings during assessment.

References

> **Questions**
>
> 1. Consider this chapter's content and apply what you have learnt to a recent patient.
> 2. Thinking about this patient, did they have any frailty syndromes, polypharmacy, reduced function that challenged your treatments?
> 3. How do the theories of ageing affect your assessment for major trauma?

Further Resources

- Banerjee J et al. (2017). *Major trauma in older people. Trauma Audit and Research Network (TARN)*. Available at: https://www.researchgate.net/publication/317030697_Major_Trauma_in_Older_People
- General BroadCAST podcast. (n.d.). *Silver trauma episode*. Available at: https://www.generalbroadcast.org.uk/blog/silver-trauma
- MDTea podcast series. (n.d.). *Series 7, Episode 2 – Silver trauma*. Available at: https://thehearingaidpodcasts.org.uk/mdtea-podcast/
- Raven D (2019). *HECTOR: The Heartlands' Elderly Care Trauma and Ongoing Recovery Programme*. Available at: https://www.embeds.co.uk/wp-content/uploads/2019/10/Hector-manual.pdf

References

Alqarni AG, et al. (2023). Does frailty status predict outcome in major trauma in older people? A systematic review and meta-analysis. *Age and Ageing*, 52(5): afad073.

Criado Perez C (2019). *Invisible Women: Exposing data bias in a world designed for men*. London: Chatto and Windus.

Dixon J, et al. (2019). Age and the distribution of major injury across a national trauma system. *Age and Ageing*, 49(2): 218–226.

Dixon J, et al. (2022). Regional variation in the provision of major trauma services for the older injured patient. *Injury*, 53(7): 2470–2477.

Joint Royal Colleges Ambulance Liaison Committee (JRCALC) and Association of Ambulance Chief Executives (AACE) (2022). *JRCALC Clinical Guidelines 2022*. Bridgwater: Class Professional Publishing.

Kehoe A, et al. (2015). The changing face of major trauma in the UK. *Emergency Medicine Journal*, 32(12): 911–915.

Kehoe A, et al. (2016). Older patients with traumatic brain injury present with a higher GCS score than younger patients for a given severity of injury. *Emergency Medicine Journal*, 33(6): 381–385.

National Institute for Health and Care Excellence (2016a). Major trauma: assessment and initial management (NICE guideline NG39). Available at: https://www.nice.org.uk/guidance/ng39/evidence/full-guideline-2308122833 [accessed 28th September 2023].

National Institute for Health and Care Excellence (2016b). Hip fracture in adults NICE quality standard. Available at: https://www.nice.org.uk/guidance/qs16/documents/draft-quality-standard-2#:~:text=About%2070%2C000%20to%2075%2C000%20hip,is%20about%20%C2%A32%20billion [accessed 27th September 2023].

Nicholson H, et al. (2022). Factors influencing conveyance of older adults with minor head injury by paramedics to the emergency department: a multiple methods study. *BMC Emergency Medicine*, 22(1): 184.

Raven D (2019). HECTOR: The Heartlands' elderly care trauma & ongoing recovery programme. Available at: https://www.embeds.co.uk/wp-content/uploads/2019/10/Hector-manual.pdf [accessed 2nd September 2023].

Trauma Audit and Research Network (TARN) (2017). England and Wales. Major trauma in older people. Available at: https://aacesite.s3.eu-west-2.amazonaws.com/wp-content/uploads/2017/04/04105743/Major-Trauma-in-Older-People-2017.pdf [accessed 28th May 2024].

Chapter 10

Palliative and End-of-Life Care

Edward O'Brian

Learning Points

By the end of this chapter, you will:

- Understand the difference between palliative and end-of-life care
- Understand the components of a holistic assessment and the concept of total pain
- Recognise indicators suggestive that a person may have an end-of-life care need
- Recognise the dying patient
- Understand the common symptoms at the end of life and their management.

Case Study

Background: You are responding to a 999 call in a care home for Stan, a 75-year-old man who has COPD and low sats.

Presenting Complaint: Stan is very breathless; the care home staff noted his oxygen saturations to be 88% on O_2 and therefore called 999.

History of Complaint: The staff member reports that Stan has deteriorated gradually over time. His breathing is no worse today in presentation than it has been in the last week or so, but as his oxygen saturations are lower today than previously, the staff member has called 999. Although talking is a struggle, the patient is clear that he does not want to attend hospital.

Past Medical History: COPD. Has oxygen concentrator running 24/7.

Allergies: None known.

CHAPTER 10 Palliative and End-of-Life Care

Drug History: Oxygen, multiple inhalers including salbutamol, tiotropium bromide and umeclidinium. Steroids, antibiotics. Diazepam.

Social History

Lives in a care home. Requires assistance with ADLs. Has a daughter from a previous marriage who lives far away, she visits once a month. Patient is happy for any information to be shared with her if needed.

Assessment

- **GCS score:** 15 (E4/V5/M6)
- **Heart rate:** 110 irregular bpm
- **Blood pressure:** 109/78
- **Blood glucose:** 7.9 mmols
- **Respiratory rate:** 36 breaths per minute
- **Oxygen saturations:** 86%
- **Temperature:** 37.5°C
- **Frailty score:** CFS score 9

Holistic Assessment

Physical

Breathing: Marked breathlessness. Unable to walk short distance from chair to bathroom due to increase in breathlessness. Constant wheeze. Basal crackles on auscultation. Unable to complete sentences.

Pain: Denies pain.

Nausea and Vomiting: Denies nausea or vomiting.

Oral Intake/Oral Health: Poor oral intake, loss of appetite over weeks with new dysphagia reported. Mouth appears dry. No evidence of candida.

Bowel Function: Denies constipation, some loose stools but on antibiotics for last few weeks.

Urinary Function: Reduced urine output. Urine appears dark.

Fatigue: Sleeping on and off throughout day, reports feeling 'worn out'.

Sleep Pattern: Sleeping in chair at night. Has night sedation to improve sleep quality.

Communication: Good vision/hearing.

Cognition: Oriented to place, time and person. No confusion noted.

Psychological

Emotional: No issues raised, patient accepting of his fate and recognises time is likely short. No apparent fear or depression evident.

Mood: Stable.

Interests: Enjoys watching films on television.

Anxiety: Appears anxious, likely due to severe breathlessness.

Spiritual

No religious beliefs or areas of support identified. No anger identified.

Impression: End-stage COPD. Has been deteriorating for months, deterioration now evident week by week. Patient presenting as sick enough to die. Likely within his last weeks of life.

Treatment Plan

Non-Pharmacological Measures

Positioning, use of pillows on chair to keep patient sat upright. Ensure room temperature is appropriate; being too hot will increase breathlessness. Advise on the use of fan therapy for breathlessness. Request air-filled cushion for seat to reduce the risk of pressure injuries.

Pharmacological Measures

Oxygen (already on own). Nebuliser – ambulance service nebuliser (salbutamol then ipratropium bromide). Morphine for breathlessness if appropriate but consider shared decision making first.

Shared Decision Making

The decision to administer Oramorph® or morphine sulfate subcutaneously (if available on the ambulance) should be with the clinician overseeing the patient's care, for example their GP, Macmillan, in home hospice care or the community team. Discuss cessation of routine observations by the care home staff as burden likely outweighs benefit. Observations are likely to continue to deteriorate. Request the prescribing of Oramorph and just in case (JIC) medications and follow-up. Explain to care home staff that time is likely short and focus should therefore be on comfort measures.

Using communication skills, find out the patient's understanding of his current condition: find out what he may want to know, if he wants to know about prognosis, share with him that time is likely short. Reassure him that we will do all we can to make him comfortable. Ask Stan if he would like information shared with his daughter, if so, consider doing this or asking care home to do this (if she visits monthly, she may wish to visit sooner).

CHAPTER 10 Palliative and End-of-Life Care

Introduction

Ambulance services in the UK respond frequently to patients who are at the end of their life due to a terminal or advanced illness. A study by the Welsh Ambulance Services University NHS Trust (WAST) analysed deaths of the population of Wales between 2016 and 2019, specifically looking at patients with a palliative condition who accessed unscheduled care and 999 in their last 12 months of life (Secure Anonymised Information Linkage [SAIL] Databank Data, 2023). The results highlighted that on average 9% of WAST's incidents each year are to respond to a patient in the last 12 months of their life due to a palliative condition. To give that number perspective, major trauma, which many would likely associate as being more typical ambulance service work, is around 2% of WAST incidents each year.

On average 81% of deaths per year in Wales relate to a palliative condition, with an average 55% of that number being a person aged 80 years and over (SAIL Data, 2023). From this data it is reasonable to conclude that a high number of ambulance service 999 calls to support a patient at the end of their life will be related to frailty. While this data is specific to Wales, it is likely that this trend will be replicated across all UK ambulance services.

Advancing frailty is often not recognised nor is it planned for, resulting in calls to the ambulance service for a 'sudden deterioration', when in fact the sudden deterioration was likely predictable many weeks or months prior to the crisis event that triggered the 999 call. Late recognition can impede both the choice of a person's place of care, as well as restrict patient-centred decisions. This may then lead to inappropriate lifesaving interventions and the under-treatment of palliative symptoms and concerns (BGS, 2020).

Palliative and End-of-Life Care

Palliative care is for people who are living with an advanced condition or a terminal illness and where a cure is not possible. Some common conditions may include advanced frailty, dementia, cancer, heart failure and COPD.

Palliative care provides a holistic approach to a person's care, meaning it focuses not just on symptom control, which may include non-pharmacological and pharmacological intervention, but on helping people to live well until they die. How this looks may differ from person to person. In addition to clinical or physical support, palliative care also focuses on a person's spiritual, psychological and social support needs.

Physical support seeks to manage a person's symptoms, such as pain or breathlessness. It also aims to prevent additional symptoms from presenting, such as constipation due to opioids. Support from allied health professionals may also be offered such as a palliative occupational therapist or physiotherapist to help improve a person's quality of life.

Spiritual support, which may or may not include religious support, seeks to help a person with any anger they may feel because of their palliative condition. A person may question why this is happening to them: the 'why me?' question. The person may be fearful of what may happen to them as their disease or condition progresses. It may also trigger a loss of faith, as they struggle to find meaning in their situation.

Psychological support is provided when a person is experiencing symptoms such as anxiety, low mood or depression because of their palliative condition. For example, they may fear that they will suffer as their illness progresses which may cause anxiety and lead to feelings of hopelessness.

Social support may include assistance with any financial concerns. It can also help a person who has worries surrounding the family that will be left behind after their death. Social support can be helpful when a person feels a loss of role or social status, or perhaps a loss of role within the family.

A holistic assessment will likely be undertaken when a person begins to receive palliative care, however it is also something that should be considered when supporting a palliative patient who presents with pain. Using a holistic approach addresses a person's 'total pain', as illustrated in Figure 10.1. While a person may need analgesia for their physical pain, analgesia will not help the patient who is feeling psychological pain from their fear of suffering or spiritual pain from their anger towards their health. Psychological, spiritual and social pain can all further exacerbate a person's physical pain.

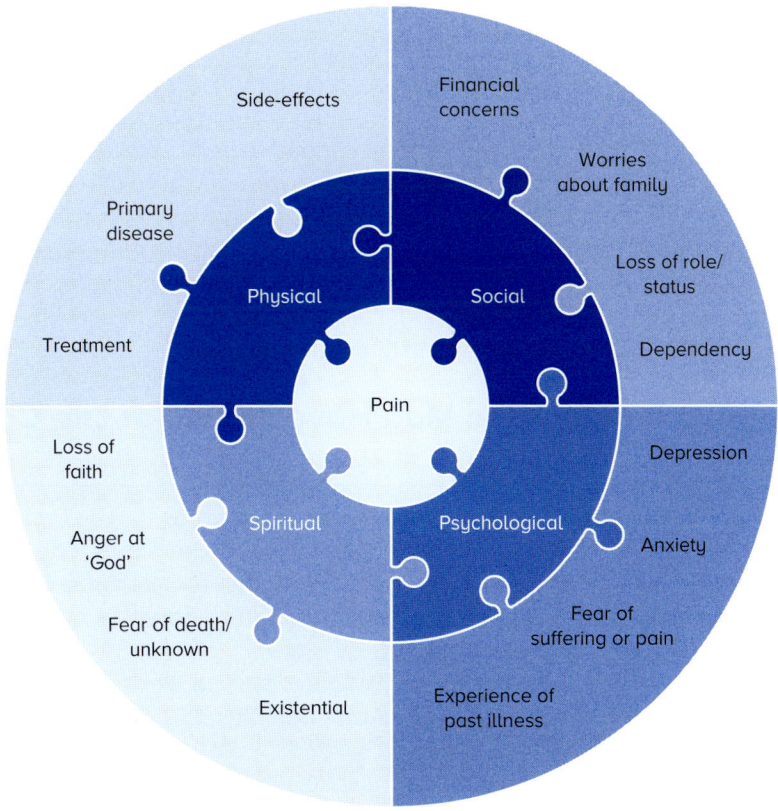

Figure 10.1 Total pain.

CHAPTER 10 Palliative and End-of-Life Care

End-of-life care is a term used when a person with a palliative condition is considered to be in their last 12 months of life (NICE, 2020). Predicting when someone may die can be very difficult, so although 12 months is widely recognised as being the definition for end-of-life care, for some, it may not be until their last months or weeks of life that end-of-life care is delivered.

End-of-life care, similar to palliative care, seeks to manage a person's symptoms and provide holistic care. End-of-life care may involve an increase in physical support, such as assistance with personal care and feeding. The person may no longer be mobile, therefore a hospital style bed may be provided in their home and a POC put in place.

In summary, all patients receiving end-of-life care are palliative care patients, but not all palliative care patients are end-of-life care patients.

Advance Care Planning

Advance care planning, a term that describes an ongoing conversation between a person and their care provider, is part of end-of-life care. Advance care planning seeks to ensure a person's wishes are met wherever possible. This may include what the person would or would not want their care to look like as they become more unwell, a discussion of their preferred place of care (PPC) and their preferred place of death (PPD) and ceilings of treatment where appropriate. A ceiling of treatment is a term used to describe when a person or their care provider believes that an intervention or treatment would deliver more burden than benefit. The process of advance care planning may then be captured and summarised in an advance care plan. An older adult who has received a diagnosis of dementia, for example, may wish to record on their advance care plan where their PPC and PPD is. As their condition then progresses, and they are no longer able to share this, care providers will be aware of where that person would or would not want to be cared for. There are many different advance care plan templates used throughout the UK, but all are there to share the patient's preferences with a care provider at a time when the patient can no longer voice those preferences. While an advance care plan is not legally binding, the information contained within should always be considered when making a best interests decision for a patient.

Recognising a Patient Who May Have an End-of-Life Care Need

Recognising an older person with deteriorating health, such as in the context of advanced frailty or an older adult with multiple advanced conditions, can help them and their care provider to plan ahead. It enables a person to give consideration as to what they may or may not want with regards to their future care.

General indicators that may help to identify an older person who is approaching the end of their life include the following (Nicholson et al., 2018):

- Two or more unplanned hospital admissions in the past 6–12 months
- Persistent and recurrent infections

- Weight loss of 5–10% in the past 6 months
- Multiple morbidity in addition to frailty
- Combined frailty and dementia
- Delirium
- Exacerbation of falling
- Rapidly rising frailty score
- Escalating patient, family or service provider distress
- Older person asking for palliative care support and/or withdrawal of active treatment.

The Gold Standards Framework (GSF) prognostic indicator lists three triggers that suggest that a person is nearing the end of their life (Thomas, 2011):

1. The surprise question: 'would you be surprised if this patient were to die in the next few months, weeks or days?'
2. General indicators of decline: deterioration, increasing need or choice for no further care.
3. Specific clinical indicators related to certain conditions.

While general indicators of decline can be similar across a few different conditions, specific clinical indicators may be unique to certain conditions. For example, in patients with cancer, metastatic cancer (meaning the cancer has spread to other parts of the body) is a specific clinical indicator that a cancer patient may have an end-of-life care need. For patients with COPD, fulfilling the criteria for long-term oxygen therapy and having more than six weeks of steroids in the preceding six months is a specific clinical indicator that a COPD patient may have an end-of-life care need (Thomas, 2011).

To help recognise a patient who may have an end-of-life care need, it is useful to familiarise yourself with The Gold Standards Framework Prognostic Indicator (Thomas, 2011) or the Supportive and Palliative Care Indicators Tool (SPICT) (University of Edinburgh, 2022). Both are freely accessible online.

Recognising the Dying Patient

Accurately predicting in advance when someone will die is extremely difficult due to the unpredictability of advanced conditions and, at best, it can really only be a guess based on the patient's speed of deterioration.

It is not uncommon for a relative to ask the question of 'how long have they got left?'. There is no magic formula for working this out, but there are indicators to help us recognise the dying patient and to help us estimate an approximate prognosis. Twycross and Wilcock state,

CHAPTER 10 Palliative and End-of-Life Care

'as a rough guide one way to look forward is to look back and consider how things have been changing. If things have been getting worse month by month, perhaps we are talking about planning ahead a few months at a time. If things have been changing week by week, maybe we are talking about planning a few weeks at a time and if day by day maybe take things a few days at a time'

(Twycross and Wilcock, 2016).

This guide is often used by clinicians working within specialist palliative care, as a patient's speed of deterioration will often be an indicator as to their prognosis where no reversible cause is apparent. So, a patient that is deteriorating and becoming more unwell week by week may be in their last weeks of life, or a patient that is deteriorating day by day may be in their last days of life.

Reviewing a person's pattern of deterioration can help when weighing up if deterioration is likely related to progression of their condition, or if a reversible cause should be suspected. Good history taking is one of your primary tools in helping you do this. A patient that was mobilising and out shopping yesterday, but today is unrousable in bed is far more likely to have a potentially reversible condition than a patient who has been progressively deteriorating over weeks. It is also helpful to consider if the patient is following their likely disease trajectory.

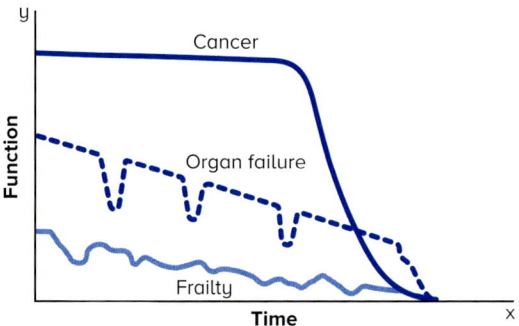

Figure 10.2 Illness trajectories and palliative care.

Figure 10.2 depicts the typical disease trajectory from diagnosis to death for common palliative conditions. The y-axis represents the patient's function, with 'high function' indicating the patient is still active, so they may be able to do their own shopping or go on holiday, for example. 'Low function' would indicate that the patient may require assistance with the likes of washing and dressing, or they may be bed-bound.

The x-axis represents time, with the left side of the graph being point of diagnosis and the right-side being death.

The line denoted as 'cancer' shows how a patient can live well for a period, however, once deterioration commences, the decline can be rapid. This sharp drop in function may be months to weeks, however in some cases this may even be weeks to days.

Organ failure may be a heart failure or a COPD patient, for example. At the point of diagnosis, the graph highlights that this group of patients are less likely to be as high functioning as a typical cancer patient is at diagnosis. The disease trajectory for this group of patients can often follow a different pattern, one that has sudden deterioration episodes, but episodes that can be managed to help improve function. You will note from the graph, however, that the improvement will not get the patient back to the level they were prior to their deterioration. There are often multiple episodes of a sudden drop in function and, despite intervention improving the patient's symptoms, the overall pattern is still one of continuous deterioration.

The frailty line shows that the function is low and continues to decline. As an ambulance clinician responding to a 999 call for a patient who is in this category and who is nearing the end of their life, the information offered by a relative or carer may be that the patient has experienced a sudden deterioration. Good history taking will help to determine if this is in fact a sudden deterioration or if they are deteriorating as a result of their advanced condition.

Key Assessment Questions

Was the patient fully mobile or washing, dressing and feeding themself yesterday? If so, it may well be a sudden deterioration and therefore a potential reversible cause. Or, has the patient been deteriorating over the last months, weeks and days? Have they become increasingly frail? Has their mobility deteriorated? Are they sleeping more? Has their appetite been declining and are they having trouble with their swallow recently? If it was yes to all, perhaps it is not a sudden deterioration, perhaps they are following the disease trajectory that we would expect to see in a dying patient. Gathering detailed information on how the patient has been over the past months, weeks, and days, combined with an understanding of disease trajectories, is crucial for assessing their condition.

Shared Decision Making

It can be very helpful for ambulance clinicians managing an end-of-life care situation to carry out shared decision making with a senior clinician (alongside the patient, if able, and their family). JRCALC guidelines specific to end-of-life care state,

> 'in managing end of life situations, where there may be a need to administer medicines for symptom control or facilitate the patient's preference with regard to the place of care, remember that the patient's existing care team will hold more information about them and have met them in person in the past. Shared decision making by contacting and discussing cases with the patient's General Practitioner, an out of hours General Practitioner or local palliative care team is invaluable'
>
> (JRCALC and AACE 2022).

Difficult Conversations

Chapter 2: Person-Centred Communication outlines taking a holistic approach that takes into consideration the life of the patient and the biases of the clinician. During encounters with patients at the end of life or who are receiving palliative treatment, conversations can be difficult for both the provider and the patient, their family, relatives and carers.

Conversations should be tailored to the patient, using simple language with no jargon. Where required, adjust according to their level of understanding and use the services of trusted interpreters or interpreting services. Be clear with the message being relayed, but also ensure you check for understanding. It is good practice to document the conversation had, who was there and your impression of how the message was understood. As the 2014 Marie Curie exploration of difficult conversations observes, not initiating conversations about what people want, expect and understand can create problems for all involved.

Common Symptoms in End-of-Life Care and Their Management

While it is not uncommon for a person in their last months of life to experience symptoms such as hiccups, itching or oral problems like a dry mouth or candidosis (oral thrush), these common symptoms are less likely to trigger a 999 call.

Many patients who are suspected to be in their last months, weeks or days of life will be prescribed just in case or anticipatory medications. These medications are kept in the person's care setting for use by a doctor, nurse or paramedic. These medications will likely include analgesia for pain, an anti-emetic for nausea and vomiting, an anxiolytic for agitation and an anti-secretory for respiratory secretions.

The five common symptoms which are more likely to trigger a 999 call, and therefore require an emergency response, are listed below along with suggested management techniques.

Pain

Pain, along with breathlessness, is the most common symptom experienced by a person at the end of life. Around 80% of patients with cancer and 67% of patients with cardiovascular disease or COPD will experience moderate to severe pain at end of life (WHO, 2023).

Chronic pain related to a person's condition is termed background pain. This will likely be managed with regular analgesia. A person may also be prescribed additional analgesia for breakthrough pain. Breakthrough pain is a term used to describe when a person's background pain increases compared to their normal level of pain and may require a dose of analgesia when required on top of their background analgesia.

In order to help manage a patient's pain effectively, we first need to understand the likely cause of the pain. There will be occasions when a clinician is asked to manage a patient who is displaying signs of being in pain, but that person is not able to communicate where their pain is, perhaps due to dementia or a loss of capacity. In addition to physical pain, total pain, as described earlier in the chapter, should always be considered as a potential cause or aggravating factor.

Common Symptoms in End-of-Life Care and Their Management

Non-Pharmacological Management

With a non-pharmacological approach to pain management, especially when assessing the likely cause of physical pain in someone who cannot communicate it, such as an older adult with advanced dementia, it is important to consider the person's positioning. As a person becomes more poorly, they will likely spend longer periods of time in bed; this leaves the person susceptible to developing pressure sores. Common areas to develop pressure injuries are the which a person's weight is transferred to when in prolonged lying and/or seated positions. This may include the back of the head, shoulders, elbows, back and coccyx area. It may also include the back of the knees, their heels or their hips. Asking the person who is caring for the patient how often they are being turned or if they have any known pressure areas may help to indicate if pressure injuries may be a cause of the patient's pain, and where a pressure injury is suspected, consideration should be given to exposing and examining the person's skin. If the patient is lying on a pressure injury, turning them so they are no longer lying on it may be all that is required to manage their pain.

In addition to pressure injuries, consideration should be given to urine retention and/or constipation as a possible cause of a person's pain. Again, ask the person caring for the patient for information. Has the patient passed urine or opened their bowels recently? Consider an abdominal examination, to include visualisation for distention, palpation and listening for bowel sounds using a stethoscope.

Pharmacological Management

Opioids are the mainstay of pain control in end-of-life care (Platt, 2010). A patient may already be taking morphine in the form of tablets, liquid or via a syringe driver. Where pain is intense and opioids are already prescribed, morphine should be the first line treatment for breakthrough pain (JRCALC and AACE, 2022). When morphine cannot be given, perhaps due to sensitivity or renal function problems, oxycodone is commonly prescribed. This has the same therapeutic effect but is metabolised via the liver as opposed to the kidneys.

If a person has just in case or anticipatory medications prescribed, the analgesia and dose on the drug chart should be favoured over the use of ambulance service analgesia: this is because the patient's medication is tailored to them and therefore more likely to be effective. Pain in a dying patient is an emergency and cannot be left untreated.

Breathlessness

Breathlessness, as the other most common symptom at the end of life alongside pain, is present in 90% of patients at some point during the last 3 days of life (Rogers et al., 2023).

When managing a person with breathlessness, if hypoxia is not present, then oxygen is not indicated. Remember, oxygen is a cure for hypoxia, it is not a cure for breathlessness.

Breathlessness may be a secondary response to another symptom. For example, a person in pain may also appear breathless due to their pain. Managing that person's pain may help reduce their breathlessness.

Breathlessness can be common in patients with lung function problems, such as lung cancer or COPD. Where lung function problems are not known to be present, other causes of breathlessness can include limb and respiratory muscle weakness related to a person's physical frailty or cachexia (Twycross et al., 2016).

When assessing a breathless patient, history taking will help determine why they may be breathless and if there are any potential reversible causes. Gather information to ascertain how long they have been breathless for. Are there any aggravating factors, such as exertion, or is the person breathless at rest? Assess the person's anxiety and/or pain levels to see if this may be triggering their breathlessness. Are there any social or psychological influences? When examining the patient, is central cyanosis present? Do they have a new onset of high temperature? Where possible, auscultate the chest: are the breath sounds equal? is there good air entry? For some patients a potential reversible cause such as an infection or a pleural effusion may be present. However, for many patients, breathlessness will be part of their physical condition and the focus should be on good symptom management.

Non-Pharmacological Management

Non-pharmacological management of breathlessness includes positioning – if a patient is lying flat, sitting them up may bring relief. A person sitting up in a chair who is breathless may find it helpful to lean forward and rest their elbows on their knees. Pursed lip breathing whereby a person inhales through the nose and then exhales slowly through pursed lips may help relieve the experience of breathlessness.

Use of fan therapy can be very helpful in relieving breathlessness. Encourage the person to hold a handheld fan at approximately 15 cm in front of the face. When air passes across the receptors on the face that are situated around the mouth and nose, this sends a signal to the brain that reduces the sensation of breathlessness (NHS Highland, 2019).

Pharmacological Management

Pharmacological management of breathlessness will primarily involve using opioids, such as liquid morphine for self-administration, or morphine which is administered subcutaneously or intramuscularly in low doses. In instances where morphine cannot be tolerated, oxycodone liquid may be self-administered, or oxycodone may be prescribed in injectable form. Benzodiazepines may also be prescribed to patients to help relieve breathlessness; this is particularly helpful when anxiety or agitation is also a factor.

Anxiety and Agitation

Anxiety and agitation are not dissimilar, but how the patient presents for each may differ slightly. Anxiety tends to present as a fear, whereas agitation may lead to a person displaying frustration or anger. While some anxiety may be considered a natural response to life-limiting illness, it is important to identify and treat the exaggerated response which is classified as pathological anxiety (Palliative Care Guidelines, 2012). Anxiety often stems from uncertainty, fear about the future and separation from loved ones (Twycross et al., 2016). For some, anxiety or agitation may be long term; it may pre-date their current condition. Others may have a long-term history of addiction, such as smoking. If their condition or illness is now preventing them from smoking, nicotine withdrawal may be a trigger for agitation.

Managing anxiety and agitation may require the management of a combination of causes, so good history taking will be key to understanding potential causes. If pain or breathlessness is present, this may well trigger anxiety or agitation, therefore managing the pain and/or breathlessness may reduce the anxiety or agitation. Symptoms may be medication-related: asking about any new medications or recent dose changes to current medications may be useful.

Non-Pharmacological Management

Finding out when a person last passed urine or opened their bowels is important, particularly if that person is not able to communicate. A full bladder, as a result of urine retention for example, would very likely lead to a person displaying agitation. Infection should also be considered as a possible trigger for a new anxiety or agitation.

When managing anxiety and agitation, effective communication is important. Explain to the patient who you are and what your role is; provide reassurance to that person and involve friends, family or carers. Environmental factors should be considered. A person lying in a bed feeling anxious will likely feel more anxious if you stand at the foot of the bed towering over them to ask questions. Consider your own position and, where possible, match your height to their height. So, for the person in bed, kneeling or sitting next to them, so that you are at eye level with them, will be less intimidating. Also consider other environmental factors such as lighting or background noise, an anxious person in a room with low-level lighting and shadows may feel less anxious if the room is well lit.

Pharmacological Management

Pharmacological management of anxiety or agitation will often be through benzodiazepines such as lorazepam tablets for self-administration. When a person is nearing the end of their life and experiencing agitation, often referred to as terminal agitation, this may require injectable medication such as midazolam to help them settle.

Nausea and Vomiting

Nausea is an unpleasant feeling of the need to vomit often accompanied by autonomic symptoms. Vomiting is the forceful expulsion of gastric contents through the mouth (Twycross et al., 2016).

Continued nausea can be extremely debilitating and have a negative psychological effect on a person. Nausea may be accompanied by cold sweats, diarrhoea

CHAPTER 10   Palliative and End-of-Life Care

and tachycardia. Management of nausea and vomiting will often require a pharmacological approach due to limited non-pharmacological options.

Non-Pharmacological Management

Dietary advice such as advising a person to sip drinks slowly or to only eat small amounts can be helpful in preventing exacerbation of a person's nausea, but it is unlikely to assist in controlling the symptom in the same way that non-pharmacological approaches can help with other common symptoms.

Pharmacological Management

Management of nausea is primarily done using an injectable anti-emetic. The likely cause of a person's nausea will inform the prescriber which anti-emetic is most likely to be effective, therefore if a person has a prescribed anti-emetic in their home as part of their just in case or anticipatory medications, using that should be favoured over an anti-emetic that is carried by the ambulance or employing community service.

As a guide to understanding why a person may have a specific anti-emetic prescribed, metoclopramide is likely to be prescribed for gastric stasis or compression. Cyclizine can be helpful for motion sickness, bowel obstruction or raised intracranial pressure. Levomepromazine is more of a broad-spectrum anti-emetic so useful when the cause is not certain, and haloperidol can be effective in treating medication-related nausea or bio-chemical abnormalities.

It is worth remembering that an anti-emetic is designed to reduce or stop a person from feeling sick; it will not stop a person from vomiting if there is something to expel. So, if a person has had nausea and vomiting and they are then administered an anti-emetic, they no longer feel nauseous, but they have an episode of vomiting, the anti-emetic has worked. It has stopped that person experiencing the very unpleasant psychological sensation of nausea, which can often be far worse than the physical experience of vomiting.

Respiratory Secretions

The noise created by respiratory secretions can often lead to panic and fear for those looking after a dying patient. The sound may lead care givers to fear the patient may be choking or drowning, leading them to call 999.

Respiratory secretions are a strong predictor that time is likely short as they are mostly heard in the last days or hours of a person's life. A person will probably be sleeping and unrousable at the time respiratory secretions are heard; they will not be awake or communicating at this point (Marie Curie, 2022).

We produce on average around 750 millilitres of saliva in a 24-hour period, but we swallow this throughout the day without giving it any thought. A person in their last hours of life will no longer be swallowing their saliva as they would have done previously, as swallow problems and generalised weakness, which limit the ability to cough and clear the throat, are likely to be present at this stage. As the person is likely to be lying flat in bed at this stage, saliva can pool in the throat. Where this pooling occurs, as the person breaths, air passes through and creates a bubbling or rattling sound, similar to what would happen if you blew down a straw into a cup of water. As the pooling is near the vocal cords the bubbling noise is amplified, making it sound worse than it is. Essentially, respiratory secretions are a little bit of fluid in a very noisy place.

Non-Pharmacological Management

Respiratory secretions are very unlikely to cause the patient any pain or distress and so reassurance and explanation to those supporting the patient should be the primary focus. Helping those present to understand that the noise is just a small pooling of saliva as the patient is too weak to clear their throat may be all that is required. Reassure them that this is not affecting their breathing or causing the person any distress. Consideration may also be given to patient positioning to allow for postural drainage, however, if the person looks comfortable, the focus should be on reassurance.

If there is no other noise in the room, those sat around the bed will not hear anything but the sound of the respiratory secretions. Asking a family member or loved one if the patient likes listening to the radio or some music can sometimes be an effective distraction technique for those who still seem worried by the noise. Introducing another sound at a low-level means that the rattling or bubbling sound is no longer the only noise in the room to focus on and can help remove anxiety.

Pharmacological Management

Pharmacological management of respiratory secretions will often not be necessary if the non-pharmacological methods have been effective. There is also very poor evidence to support the use of anti-secretory medication such as hyoscine hydrobromide or glycopyrronium (Bennett et al., 2002). Where an anti-secretory is used it may prevent build-up of further secretions, but it will not dry up any secretions already present.

Conclusion

A high number of 999 calls to ambulance services across the UK involve older adults with a chronic medical condition. This includes adults who have deteriorated as a result of their ongoing worsening health, but may not have been 'labelled' as palliative at the time of the 999 call. A common example of this may be an older adult with advanced frailty. The 999 call may not specifically be for a deterioration, it may be because of a fall. The next time you respond to an older adult, think about the 'Recognising a patient who may have an end-of-life care need' section above. Looking out for these signs will help us to better identify a person who may have an end-of-life care need. Sharing our thoughts with colleagues in community and primary care (where appropriate) can then help to ensure advance care planning can take place earlier, which in turn helps to ensure a person has more choice about the future direction of their care.

CHAPTER 10 Palliative and End-of-Life Care

> **Questions**
>
> 1. Consider this chapter's content and apply what you have learnt to a recent patient.
> 2. Thinking about this patient, did you feel confident managing this situation?
> 3. What resources are available to assist you with difficult decisions? Who is your MDT when faced with a dying patient?

Further Resources

- Further reading on palliative and end-of-life care can be found on websites hosted by charity organisations such as Macmillan or Marie Curie. Typing 'what is palliative care' into your web browser will bring up lots of useful resources.
- Macmillan (2024). *Palliative and end of life care*. Available at: https://www.macmillan.org.uk/coronavirus/healthcare-professionals/palliative-and-end-of-life-care
- Marie Curie (2014). *Difficult conversations with dying people and their families*. Available at: https://www.mariecurie.org.uk/globalassets/media/documents/s691-difficult-conversations-report.pdf
- Marie Curie (2022). *What is palliative care?* Available at: https://www.mariecurie.org.uk/help/support/diagnosed/recent-diagnosis/palliative-care-end-of-life-care

Acknowledgements

The editors would like to thank Kieran Potts, Senior Research Fellow, North West Ambulance Services NHS Trust for his initial contribution to this chapter.

References

Bennett M, et al. (2002). Using anti-muscarinic drugs in the management of death rattle: evidence-based guidelines for palliative care. *Palliative Medicine*, 16(5): 369–374.

British Geriatrics Society (BGS) (2020). End of life care in frailty: identification and prognostication. Available at: https://www.bgs.org.uk/resources/end-of-life-care-in-frailty-identification-and-prognostication [accessed 28th May 2024].

Joint Royal Colleges Ambulance Liaison Committee (JRCALC) and Association of Ambulance Chief Executives (AACE) (2022). *JRCALC Clinical Guidelines 2022*. Bridgwater, UK: Class Professional Publishing.

Marie Curie (2022). Noisy chest secretions towards the end of life. Available at: https://www.mariecurie.org.uk/professionals/palliative-care-knowledge-zone/symptom-control/noisy-secretions#:~:text=In%20the%20last%20days%20of%20a%20person%27s%20life%2C%20secretions%20(fluid,called%20%27the%20death%20rattle%27 [accessed 28th May 2024].

Murray SA, et al. (2005). Illness trajectories and palliative care. *British Medical Journal*, 330(7498): 1007–1011.

References

National Institute for Health and Care Excellence (NICE) (2020). End of life care for adults. Available at: https://www.nice.org.uk/about/what-we-do/into-practice/measuring-the-use-of-nice-guidance/impact-of-our-guidance/nice-impact-end-of-life-care-for-adults [accessed 28th May 2024].

NHS Highland (2019). Managing breathlessness. Available at: https://patientinfo.nhshighland.scot.nhs.uk/Respiratory/Handheld%20fan.pdf [accessed 15th August 2023].

Nicholson C, et al. (2018). What are the main palliative care symptoms and concerns of older people with multimorbidity? A comparative cross-sectional study using routinely collected phase of illness, Australia-modified Karnofsky Performance Status and Integrated Palliative Care Outcome Scale data. *Annals of Palliative Medicine*, 7(Suppl 3): S164–S175.

Palliative Care Guidelines (2012). Available at: https://www.pallcare.info [accessed 3rd August 2023].

Platt M (2010). Pain challenges at the end of life – pain and palliative care collaboration. *Reviews in Pain*, 2010; 4(2): 18–23.

Rogers JB, Modi P, Minteer JF (2023). Dyspnea in palliative care. Available at: https://www.ncbi.nlm.nih.gov/books/NBK526122/#:~:text=It%20is%20common%20in%20many,a%20patient%20can%20distinctly%20qualify [accessed 28th May 2024].

Sail Data and Welsh Ambulance Services NHS Trust (2023). Internal data, unpublished.

Thomas K (2011). Prognostic indicator guidance (PIG) 4th edition Oct 2011. The Gold Standards Framework Centre In End of Life Care CIC. Available at: https://www.goldstandardsframework.org.uk/cd-content/uploads/files/General%20Files/Prognostic%20Indicator%20Guidance%20October%202011.pdf [accessed 28th May 2024].

Twycross R, Wilcock A (2016). *Introducing Palliative Care*. Nottingham: Palliativedrugs.com Ltd.

University of Edinburgh (2022). Supportive and Palliative Care Indicators Tool. Available at: https://www.spict.org.uk [accessed 28th May 2024].

World Health Organization (WHO) (2023). Palliative care. Available at: https://www.who.int/health-topics/palliative-care [accessed 31st July 2024].

Chapter 11

Social Care

Charlotte Walker and Peter Gosling

Learning Points

By the end of this chapter, you will:

- Understand how local authorities structure a supportive assessment for care in the home environment
- Recognise the disruption and impact on individuals requiring care and the need for shared decision making
- Value the importance of informal care givers and that this can fundamentally affect relationships.

Case Study

This case study focuses on the cared for person and as such, the clinical assessment and plan for Milly is not included. This is deliberate as we mainly concentrate on the social care factors and the impact on James.

Background: You are a paramedic working on a double crewed ambulance. You are called to a 75-year-old woman (Milly) who lives in a bungalow with her 76-year-old husband (James). The couple have four children, two nearby and two further afield. James had a stroke several years ago and Milly is James' informal carer.

The couple are retired and previously travelled and lived abroad, returning to Wales following changes in James' health. While living overseas, he had several falls which impacted on his independence and emphasised difficulties staying independent.

Incident

Milly was walking from the lounge to the bedroom at around 23:00 on a Saturday evening and slipped on a mat in the hallway. Milly injured herself and was unable to move; she shouted for help, but James did not hear her. Milly remained on the floor for seven hours. During this time James slept in his room. Milly was in severe pain, had been doubly incontinent, was cold and thirsty. Connie (Milly's sister)

CHAPTER 11 Social Care

visited following failed attempts to contact Milly and James by phone. On arrival, she immediately determined an ambulance was required as she suspected Milly had fractured her hip.

Milly has been struggling to provide informal care for her husband. Support services were previously stopped due to COVID-19 restrictions and when they restarted, they were not consistent due to the high turnover of carers. As a result, Milly was exhausted, both mentally and physically, was visibly ageing and demonstrating a reduction in her independence and ability to plan for the longer term. Milly's mental health was affected, resulting in medications being prescribed to help her mood. Before the pandemic, Milly would take James out in a disability taxi and in his converted wheelchair twice weekly, as well as having a 'sitting service' to enable her to socialise.

Assessment

Having had a severe stroke, James is unable to move his left arm and leg and his right leg. He has no ability to support his core body strength. James is aware when he needs to open his bowels or pass urine, however he is unable to do this without assistance. Mentally, James can make decisions about some of the aspects of his life and choices, but his capacity can fluctuate when he is tired or unwell. Since his stroke, James can display changing behaviours; this is usually due to frustration, leading him to call out to Milly, demanding that she undertakes certain tasks such as making tea, changing the television channel or assisting with a bottle for urinating. James had access to a day care service on a Monday morning to enable Milly a few hours respite, while James had the opportunity to interact with others and have a break from home and Milly. However, James used to refuse most weeks to attend as he felt it was not interesting and he did not like the food or being away from home. To enable James to remain at home he has domiciliary care coming in to assist him four times a day.

James' typical POC is:

> 08:00 – Carers call, assist James with toileting, washing, dressing and also make him breakfast. Carers hoist James into a specially adapted lounge chair or wheelchair. Medication is given.
>
> 12:00 – Carers call to offer to support James with pressure relief, so will offer to move him into his bed or alternate chair. Toileting and fluids provided.
>
> 17:00 – Carers call to support James with pressure relief, so they will offer to move him into his bed or alternate chair. Toileting and fluids provided.
>
> 19:30 – Carers call to wash and change James, put him into his night clothes, offer toileting and hoist James into his bed for the night.

Initial Plan

Following an assessment of James's safety, initiated by you and supported by family who remained on scene until social services arrived, it was agreed that James should access respite care at a local care home for a defined period of time.

It is hoped that, following Milly's surgery, the couple can be reunited at home. Although this is the intention, it will need to be recognised that the situation and feelings about it may have changed and it is unlikely that this will simply be a case of reinstating what was previously there.

There may have been an impact on James' care needs, having been supported in a care home environment for a number of weeks. Evidence suggests that people decondition in a hospital or a care home situation as the opportunities for self-care in a care home are extremely limited (BGS, 2017). A judgement will therefore need to be made about the level of support James will subsequently need on returning home.

A decision will need to be determined about Milly's capacity (both physically and mentally) to resume the carer role. It appears likely that, in the short term at the very least, Milly's physical health has deteriorated and that she is unlikely to be able to resume all of the caring tasks that she previously undertook, resulting in the need for additional support for James. Milly herself is going to require support in order to recover from her surgery and it is currently unclear whether she will regain full independence. Consideration will need to be given as to how to coordinate the support arrangements for both Milly and James.

Equally importantly, Milly's view of herself in the carer role may have changed. The impact of having a break from an all-consuming carer role, even if enforced, can be significant and the prospect of resuming such a role may not be one that she relishes. Being a carer, like Milly, is so all-consuming that when you have a break from it, the impact both physically and emotionally is likely to be huge. Carers in this situation will hopefully feel more rested and may have had the opportunity to glimpse life beyond that of being a carer and this may affect how they view taking the role of carer back on. This will all require careful clarification when making plans for James' return home.

Introduction

It is important from an emergency and urgent care perspective to understand the impact clinical decisions made at scene can have on the adoption, maintenance and alteration of care packages. When faced with individuals in a crisis, it is easy to see the people involved solely in the context of that crisis and to forget that, up to that point, their lives had been vastly different. It is also easy to see individuals purely in their current roles of carer and cared for. While it is understandable that the focus is on resolving the crisis, it is important that there is an appreciation of the significance of life before the crisis, as this could play a vital role in determining the best way of tackling the presenting problems. The cared for is likely to have made significant adjustments and their expectations about their own life may have changed. How successfully they have managed to make these adjustments and the impact on their self-perception and on their relationships will be relevant to how they present.

CHAPTER 11 Social Care

It will also affect their feelings about the current crisis and how it could be resolved. The working assumption should be that the patient has capacity to make decisions for themself until and unless you have substantial grounds for assuming otherwise (Mental Capacity Act 2005). This is reinforced by legal frameworks such as the Health and Social Care Act 2012 (England) and the Social Services and Well-being (Wales) Act (Social Care Wales, 2014) which have been developed to encourage individuals to have more choice in deciding what they need, while also giving them a stronger voice and control over their lives.

While there is much within this chapter that sits outside traditional urgent and emergency healthcare principles, the holistic approach to older people's care should encompass individualisation. Therefore, the following pages provide fundamental information relevant to the presentation of many older people in our communities that remain largely hidden from the paramedic workforce.

Carers and the Caring Role

Even people with a strong relationship and a well-developed sense of commitment will experience moments of doubt and frustration about the role they find themselves in. They may resent being in this role or feel that they have lost a sense of who they are. They may be angry or depressed, or they may have found strength and fulfilment in this changed role. Carers First (2021) recognise this and outline how this can create increased tension, changes in behaviour, role reversal and changes to sex and intimacy within a relationship. However, they also state the positives that come in terms of strengthening relationships through increasing positive feelings towards each partner.

Carers now have a right to an assessment of their own need for support (Care Act 2014). This is a way of understanding and recording their needs and capturing both their perceptions of the situation and what is important. Box 11.1 highlights the assessment criteria for carers from the Care Act 2014.

Box 11.1 Assessment Criteria of the Care Act 2014.

> Carers should be assessed on their:
> - Caring role and how it affects their life and well-being
> - Physical, mental and emotional health
> - Feelings and choices about caring, work, study, training and leisure
> - Relationships
> - Social activities
> - Housing
> - Planning for emergencies.

Source: based on information from Carers Wales, 2023.

Milly and James had previously had a 'sitting service' for James (a carer to sit with him) which enabled Milly to leave the home, plus respite care on occasions. Respite care is normally a short stay in a care home to allow the carer a lengthier break from caring. Day care for the cared for individual can also be an option, providing stimulation and company for the cared for individual as well as a break for the carer.

Approximately 8% of the UK's household population are informal carers and provide care estimated to equate to £57 billion (Office for National Statistics (ONS), 2017). Local authorities commission services specifically aimed at providing support to carers and it is widespread practice for services to be delivered through third sector organisations. This may come in the form of a carer's centre or hub (Cheshire East, 2024). Additionally, the offer for carers will include psychological and emotional support, plus the opportunity to share experiences, stories and coping strategies with other carers. Some authorities also offer a one-off carers grant.

Many carers find being able to talk to others in similar situations hugely helpful. The potential impact of being a carer on an individual's sense of well-being cannot be overestimated (Carers UK, 2021). This can often be just as significant a factor as the carer's physical health status. Being able to talk to others who are most likely to be able to understand a carer's lived experience, without feeling judged by family members or health and social care professionals, can be a huge help to many.

Assessment of Needs

Although it is perfectly possible for individuals to make their own care arrangements, if you are unfamiliar with social care systems and services, it can be difficult to know where to start. Many people initially contact their local authority for a list of contracted providers who deliver a quality service. This can offer families reassurance that their relative will receive known and safe levels of care. In approaching a local authority, individuals should be made aware that under the Care Act 2014 they are entitled to an assessment of their needs. Box 11.2 demonstrates the criteria local authorities should incorporate as mandated by the Care Act 2014:

Box 11.2 Criteria that Local Authorities Should Incorporate According to the Care Act 2014.

- Carry out an assessment of anyone who appears to require care and support, regardless of their likely eligibility for state-funded care
- Focus the assessment on the person's needs and how they impact on their well-being and the outcomes they want to achieve
- Involve the person in the assessment and, where appropriate, their carer or someone else they nominate
- If required provide access to an independent advocate to support involvement in the assessment
- Consider other things that can contribute to the desired outcomes (for example, preventive services or community support)
- Use the new national minimum threshold to judge eligibility for publicly funded care and support.

Source: based on information from Social Care Institute for Excellence, 2024.

CHAPTER 11 Social Care

This does not mean that the local authority is required to provide or arrange care services, but that they would complete a needs assessment with the individual requiring support and could arrange a carer's assessment if appropriate. The local authority representative (usually a social worker or social care assessor) can also discuss the options in terms of how identified needs might be met. Whatever an individual's financial situation, the local authority is also required to provide an appropriate level of support in making the agreed support service arrangements.

The Act clearly sets out that they must provide information on:

- What types of care and support are available, for example, specialised dementia care, befriending services, reablement
- The range of care and support services available to local people, that is, what the local providers offer, such as certain types of services
- What process local people need to use to get care and support that is available
- Where local people can find independent financial advice about care and support and help them to access it
- How people can raise concerns about the safety or well-being of someone who has care and support needs.

Local authorities must also help people to benefit from independent financial advice, so that individuals can get support to plan and prepare for the future costs of care. All information and advice must be provided in formats that help people to understand, regardless of their needs.

When undertaking an assessment of needs, specific information is required to determine the appropriate outcomes. Information required includes how an individual manages and maintains nutrition, personal hygiene, toileting needs, clothing, a safe and habitable environment, accessing and engaging in work, training, education or volunteering, use of essential services, local transport and facilities and if they have any caring responsibilities for a child. If the individual requires assistance to achieve these outcomes (either due to pain, distress, anxiety, length of time taken or causes danger to them or others) the adult is to be regarded as being unable to achieve an 'outcome' (The Care Act 2014).

The assessment should seek to capture the individual's own views and wishes and those of any carers involved. The conclusion drawn should consider the wider context of the individual or couple, in terms of their family and the community in which they live. The key to a good assessment is to draw out what is important to the individual concerned and to avoid making assumptions or giving opinions too early, resulting in support arrangements that are not only a poor fit for the individual but also more expensive or intrusive. A good assessment also identifies existing support arrangements and explores how viable or sustainable they are.

The assessment should tease out what the carer is comfortable with and prepared to do, what other support is available and seek to reach agreement with the carer and the cared for about where the gaps in support are.

Financial Assessment

Once an assessment is complete, the Care Act 2014 eligibility criteria needs to be applied. An adult's needs meet the eligibility criteria if the adult's needs arise from or are related to a physical or mental impairment or illness, they are unable to achieve two or more of the outcomes and consequently, there is, or is likely to be, a significant impact on the adult's well-being (The Care and Support (Eligibility Criteria) Regulations 2014).

The outcome of this process is an identification of the needs that the local authority will offer support with (in the form of services). The discussion with the individual and their carer should include how both eligible and non-eligible needs might be addressed with a set of support arrangements (support plan). This should encompass commissioned services, family support, carer input, equipment, privately purchased care and volunteers in a variety of combinations to enable 'personalised' or 'person-centred' care.

Financial Assessment

Local authorities can decide whether or not to charge for services, but in reality most local authorities do as they rely on this income. A local authority's charging policy will take into account an individual's income and savings and, for support at home and for a short stay in residential care, will include a calculation about what expenditure can be taken into account when working out what is a fair and reasonable charge. The overarching principle of the Care Act 2014 is that people should only be required to pay what they can afford and that a local authority's charging policy should be fair and easily understood (HM Government, 2014).

A financial assessment will:

- Include earnings, pensions, benefits and savings
- Assume that you are receiving all the benefits you are entitled to
- Consider people as individuals (not as part of a couple)
- Include disability-related expenditure (for example, higher heating costs because of a medical condition).

In relation to capital (in England 2024):

- If you have over £23,250 in capital, you will be required to meet the full cost of your care
- If you have less than £14,500, this will not be considered
- If you have between £14,500 and £23,250 a contribution will be calculated based on a sliding scale.

In Wales (in 2024), the capital limit is £24,000 and there is no lower threshold. Local authorities in Wales can only charge you a maximum of £100 (2024) per week for home care services regardless of how much you have in savings. This means that even if you have more than £24,000 in savings, you will only be charged a maximum of £100 a week and the council will cover the rest.

CHAPTER 11   Social Care

For both countries, if you are below the capital limit (of either £14,500 in England or £24,000 in Wales), the means test only looks at your income and you will only pay as much as you are assessed as being able to afford.

Note: *All figures and criteria are subject to change following publication and should be checked at the time of reading.*

Some care is free (for example, some short-term provision following a stay in hospital, commonly known as intermediate care). Within England, some local authorities have discretion about how they apply charging to care within the home. Because of these potential variations, it is always advisable for people to get independent advice about charges.

Being required to levy a charge for services provided is one of the key differences between health and social services. It is also one of the more controversial issues in adult social care. While explaining a charging policy is an essential element of the assessment process, it is difficult and a challenge that social workers often do not feel comfortable or confident about. It is also an area that individuals can have strong opinions on and can be a source of either conflict or confusion.

Choice and Control

One of the key themes of the Care Act 2014 is that people should feel in control and exercise their choice when making their own care arrangements. The reality is that, as people are usually making such arrangements in response to a crisis, they are not necessarily going to feel that 'being in control' is an accurate description in the circumstances. The intention, however, is that people feel that they engage in making the decisions about their care and support, that they are satisfied that the support being offered is the best fit for them from the options available and that they are being listened to.

Having carers coming into your home four times a day (like James and Milly) requires some considerable adjustment for both cared for and carer. Initially these are strangers within your environment, completing intimate personal care. This may feel intrusive, however relieved the carer may be for the support. There might also be an element of inconsistency in the service delivery and a difference in opinions and personalities affecting the situation. However, over time, many individuals and their carers become close and friendships blossom. Carers can make a dramatic difference to the lives of the cared for and their family and have a unique insight into their world becoming a helpful source of information in a crisis (SCIE, 2022).

In Milly and James' situation (breakdown of carer support due to hospitalisation), often immediate plans are put in place leading to the cared for person being moved. While this is often the only appropriate option, consideration should be to see if James could be supported within his home enabling opportunities to include extended family or friends to step in. Reviewing James' support plan may have provided some valuable information with contingency arrangements. Failure to consider these options may result in losing a well-established support arrangement with a provider that may not have availability when a new request is made.

The social worker may wish to discuss options with family members and take into account the psychological and emotional impact. For James, as well as having to see Milly injured, he may be concerned about losing his care package, leaving the family home and worrying about returning or moving to a care home, plus the practical concerns, such as cost, visiting schedules and medications. Time spent on this discussion can be invaluable as a rushed decision at this point can create a raft of unfamiliar problems that will need to be addressed eventually.

It can be the role of the social worker in such situations to try and provide some reassurance to the carer (so they can focus on their own needs) while trying to balance the needs and wishes of the cared for (which may not help provide the carer with the reassurance they are wanting). If such a situation has been anticipated and included in a support plan, these discussions can be considerably easier (rather like when there is a will in place when someone dies). It is vital that the voices of both parties are heard and the aim should be, wherever possible, to be available for a considered decision that people feel involved in and informed about.

Care Home Placements

While social services is not one of the emergency services, every local authority will have some capacity to respond to substantial risk or urgent situations quickly, including out of normal office hours. Emergency contact details may be included in an individual's support plan, but there is normally a local authority contact number with which health staff should be familiar. The local authority should be able to give a likely timescale for a response and will be able to discuss any options they might be able to offer. Alternatively, the patient may have a preference for a care home with which they are already familiar. The latter may be possible if it is clear that this would be in the patient's best interests but will depend in part on cost. Local authorities are not able to offer *carte blanche* in such situations without cost considerations, however they will take into account an individual's particular circumstances (for example, familiarity with a specific home and ease of access for family members).

The cost of a care home placement will depend on the arrangements the local authority has in place and on the care home being chosen. If the local authority has commissioned an 'emergency bed' for such situations, there may be no charge initially but if a bed is required for longer than 48 hours, it is likely that some level of charge will be incurred. The local authority representative should be able to provide information about charges which will take into account if this is a short stay and, therefore, individuals will continue to have household expenditure to meet.

Conclusion

In making appropriate social care plans, the process is very much like the assessment and support planning process that James and Milly (and many others) would have gone through when they first identified that they required support. The case study is based on an emergency situation, however breakdown in carer support is faced daily by primary and community care teams. Nevertheless, the same processes should be adopted regarding contacting social services and all the concerns previously

CHAPTER 11 Social Care

discussed, such as feeling in control and being involved in decision making, ensuring informed decisions and encouraging people to be as independent as possible. The potential for there to be a conflict of interest between carer and cared for is also a factor that will need to be taken into consideration. For all concerned, it is likely that this will be an iterative process, as the situation and the individual's needs evolve. These key principles, however, apply each time the cycle of assessment and support planning is applied.

> ### Questions
>
> 1. Reflect on a patient you have recently transferred to hospital who has a care package. Consider the impact on the patient and their family if the care is changed.
> 2. Thinking about this patient, how would frailty increase vulnerability?
> 3. What additional resources are available to patients and to assist you with these complex scenarios?

Further Resources

- Association of Directors of Adult Social Services (ADASS). (2024). *A voice for adult social care*. Available at: https://www.adass.org.uk
- Carers UK (n.d.). *About us: What we do*. Available at: https://www.carersuk.org/about-us/what-we-do/#:~:text=Our%20mission%20is%20to%20make,use%20innovation%20to%20improve%20services
- Department of Health and Social Care (2016). *Care Act factsheets*. Available at: https://www.gov.uk/government/publications/care-act-2014-part-1-fact sheets/care-act-factsheets
- Grobman LM (Ed.) (2012). *Days in the lives of social workers*. Charlottesville, VA: Whitehat Communications.
- Jordan M (2022). *The Essential Carer's Guide*. London: Hammersmith Health Books.
- Social Care Institute for Excellence (SCIE). (n.d.). *Website*. Available at: https://www.scie.org.uk

References

British Geriatrics Society (BGS) (2017). Deconditioning awareness. Available at: https://www.bgs.org.uk/resources/deconditioning-awareness [accessed 1st June 2024].

Care Act 2014. UK Public General Acts, c. 23. Available at: https://www.legislation.gov.uk/ukpga/2014/23/ contents/enacted [accessed 1st June 2024].

Care and Support (Eligibility Criteria) Regulations 2014. UK Draft Statutory Instruments. Available at: https://www.legislation.gov.uk/ukdsi/2014/9780111124185 [accessed 1st June 2024].

References

Carers First (2021). How your relationships can change when you become a carer. Available at: https://www.carersfirst.org.uk/help-and-advice/topics/how-your-relationships-can-change-when-you-become-a-carer/ [accessed 1st June 2024].

Carers UK (2021). State of caring 2021 report. Available at: https://www.carersuk.org/reports/state-of-caring-2021-report/ [accessed 1st June 2024].

Carers Wales (2023). Assessments: your guide to getting an assessment in Wales. Available at: https://www.carersuk.org/media/xkod0jcy/assessments-wales-april-2023-24.pdf [accessed 5th September 2024].

Cheshire East (2024). Live Well. Cheshire East carers hub (All Age Carers Hub). Available at: https://livewellservices.cheshireeast.gov.uk/Services/4387 [accessed 1st June 2024].

Health and Social Care Act 2012. UK Public General Acts, c 7. Available at: https://www.legislation.gov.uk/ukpga/2012/7/contents [accessed 30th September 2024].

Mental Capacity Act 2005. UK Public General Acts, c.9. Available at: https://www.legislation.gov.uk/ukpga/2005/9/contents [accessed 30th September 2024].

Office for National Statistics (ONS) (2017). Unpaid carers provide social care worth £57 billion. Available at: https://www.ons.gov.uk/peoplepopulationandcommunity/healthandsocialcare/healthandlifeexpectancies/articles/unpaidcarersprovidesocialcareworth57billion/2017-07-10 [accessed 1st June 2024].

Social Care Institute for Excellence (2022). Impact of COVID-19 on unpaid and family carers. Available at: https://www.scie.org.uk/care-providers/coronavirus-covid-19/commissioning/impact-on-citizens [accessed 1st June 2024].

Social Care Institute for Excellence (2024). Assessment of needs under the Care Act 2014. Available at: https://www.scie.org.uk/assessment-and-eligibility/assessment-of-needs-under-the-care-act-2014/ [accessed 5th September 2024]

Social Care Wales (2014). The Social Services and Well-being (Wales) Act 2014. Available at: https://socialcare.wales/resources-guidance/information-and-learning-hub/sswbact/overview [accessed 1st June 2024].

Chapter 12

Safeguarding

Gwenan Jones-Parry and Nikki Harvey

Learning Points

By the end of this chapter, you will:

- Understand what adult safeguarding means
- Recognise who could be at risk of harm
- Understand there are different types of abuse and what well-being means
- Understand there are legislative responsibilities in relation to safeguarding
- Appreciate the relevance of adult safeguarding in emergency and urgent care of older people.

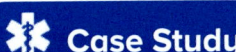 Case Study

Background: You are working as a paramedic on an ambulance responding to a call for a 70-year-old man. When you arrive, there is no way to access the property, no key safe is present and the neighbours do not have a key. You request that a family member is contacted but the neighbours have no contact numbers. In the absence of other options, you request police assistance to gain entry into the property as life status is unknown.

Once entry is gained you find sparsely furnished rooms in a state of disarray with no sign of the patient downstairs. The whole house is unclean and looks barely lived in. When you venture upstairs, you find a locked bedroom. The police gain entry into the room and you find a man, Wilf, in a state of poor personal hygiene, wearing only a soiled nappy. The room itself is void of any furniture other than a mattress on the floor which has limited bedding on it.

Presenting Complaint: Concern for welfare.

History of Presenting Complaint: Neighbours placed a 999 call for a 70-year-old man about whom they were concerned. They have not seen any signs of him in the house or any visitors to the house for a few days.

CHAPTER 12 Safeguarding

Past Medical History: Neighbours believe he has a history of mental health issues but do not know the details.

Allergies: None known.

Drug History: None known.

Social History: All the information is provided by the neighbours who called 999 and met you as you arrived. Wilf is a retired professional. He lives alone (widowed four years earlier), independently (no POC) in a semi-detached property. He has two children who visit regularly, whom the neighbours stated seem to support him. Wilf is rarely seen out and about but when he has been seen the neighbours have noticed he looks more frail and they have had increasing concerns for him in recent weeks.

Clinical Observations: These are difficult to complete as Wilf is confused and is wary of strangers. It takes time, reassurance and calm communication to complete basic clinical observations. All clinical observations lead you to believe he is dehydrated and possibly malnourished. You treat any immediate clinical concerns and keep a calm demeanour throughout to minimise any upset for the patient. Wilf does not have capacity and a best interests decision is quickly made that he requires hospitalisation for further assessment and treatment.

Impression: He is severely dehydrated, malnourished and you have significant safeguarding concerns regarding Wilf, in particular the living arrangements and his personal hygiene.

Treatment Plan: As many clinical observations as possible are completed and he is reassured. Appropriate treatment is provided in accordance with policies/procedures. One key element is to ensure Wilf is given a blanket, not only to ensure an appropriate temperature but also to maintain his dignity. He is conveyed to the nearest appropriate hospital.

Safeguarding Actions: During handover at hospital the conditions in which he was found are shared and you confirm with staff that you intend on completing a safeguarding report due to several safeguarding concerns. Police are already present on scene and they can investigate whether there are any criminal concerns.

You consider phoning the relevant adult social services team to verbally share your concerns, but decide Wilf is in no immediate danger. A safeguarding report is completed which includes all your safeguarding concerns. This safeguarding report includes information regarding the incident itself and how you came to be there, what condition Wilf was found in, where in the house he was found and all relevant environmental factors regarding his accommodation. Also included is information from his neighbours regarding his mobility and what they know regarding how he looks after himself.

Details about his support network and who within his family and friends visits and assists him would have been important to include had it been available. The report is submitted to the relevant local authority (social services) to enable further enquiries.

Safeguarding Concerns: You have several safeguarding concerns in relation to this man. You consider whether he has self-neglected to the extent it resulted in this situation, but you have significant concerns that the bedroom door was locked from the outside.

Locking the door from the outside not only restricted access to the rest of the house but also prevented egress should there be an emergency such as a fire. Had Wilf been unwell there was no access to a phone to call for assistance. His liberty had been restricted to one small bedroom.

He appeared frail and was un-clothed, dehydrated and confused when you arrived. It appeared that access to food, water and bathroom facilities was restricted. Wilf did not have access to a suitable environment, heat/warmth or anything to stimulate his mind. These factors are considered to be evidence of possible neglect by those providing care and support.

You have concerns about possible cuckooing, since Wilf had not been seen in some time and had been sequestered into one locked room, leaving the rest of the property available for misuse. Cuckooing is when the home of an adult at risk is targeted and exploited by criminals (for various criminal activities such as drug dealing).

The property, especially the bedroom he is found in, is sparsely furnished and there are concerns regarding possible financial abuse; for example, his furniture and possessions being sold.

Outcome: The local authority make enquiries, in accordance with legislation. Their enquiries reveal that Wilf's memory and mental health had deteriorated and, rather than seek further support, his family had attempted to care for him themselves. Asking for help from any organisation/charity had not been considered by them as a viable option for fear of their father being taken into a care home (which he had said before losing capacity that he did not want).

He deteriorated gradually and the family had limited his access to parts of the house as they felt this would maintain his safety. They had been struggling for months but had restricted his movements to the bedroom only for a few days prior to him being found following an incident where he had left the oven on for several days and they no longer trusted him with whole house access.

Information is gathered that Wilf's pension is still being drawn and many of his possessions have been sold. The children state that he was not using the furniture and the proceeds from the sales, along with his pension, were used to

CHAPTER 12   Safeguarding

> meet his increased care needs. His children had become overwhelmed trying to care for their father and their families at the same time as it was impacting their ability to work.
>
> While in hospital, Wilf is given an independent advocate and arrangements are put in place to meet his increased care needs. Upon hospital discharge the local authority take over the organisation and implementation of his care arrangements into the future and he returns home with a significant care package.
>
> The investigation found that there had been abuse and neglect; police investigated and decided the criminal threshold had not been met.

Introduction

Safeguarding is the protection and prevention from harm of adults at risk and children (Welsh Government, 2019). Everyone has the right to live free from harm (JRCALC and AACE, 2022). Harm is mental, physical or sexual abuse, or the impairment of social, physical, intellectual or behavioural development (Welsh Government, 2019). Adult safeguarding is a crucial part of most public services and one of the vital duties of local authorities (Ann Craft Trust (ACT), 2022). As well as reporting concerns about abuse and neglect, safeguarding also includes promoting well-being regarding all aspects of care and support (Spreadbury and Hubbard, 2020).

Safeguarding is something anyone working or volunteering with children or adults at risk of harm (adults at risk) should be aware of (Care Act 2014). Adults at risk are those with care and support needs, meaning they need assistance to enable them to live their lives. This could be due to a variety of reasons often involving financial, emotional or practical support (Starns, 2019). Practitioners working with adults at risk have a duty to recognise signs of abuse and neglect and need to know how to support and protect them by sharing their safeguarding concerns.

Safeguarding Reporting and Principles

Requirements regarding the procedures and actions for anyone working with adults at risk will be dependent upon their specific role, organisation and which UK country they work in (Starns, 2019). The mechanism for reporting safeguarding concerns varies between workplaces. All organisations have their own reporting processes, but they must have a mechanism in place to share their concerns with the relevant local authority. The local authority leads on safeguarding enquiries, but any agency can report and refer their safeguarding concerns to the local authority for consideration (Barnett, 2019).

Throughout the safeguarding process, consideration must always be given to the possibility of criminality and it may become necessary to inform or work with the police (Barnett, 2019; Dawson, 2021). Once safeguarding concerns are reported to the local authority, further enquiries will be completed to ascertain whether abuse and neglect has occurred and whether any additional actions are required (Starns, 2019). Safeguarding from significant harm is reliant upon effective professional and agency communication, co-operation and information sharing (JRCALC and AACE, 2022).

The Care Act 2014 outlines the following Adult Safeguarding Principles:

- Empowerment – enabling individuals (by encouragement and support) to give informed consent and make decisions themselves.
- Prevention – it is always beneficial to prevent harm from occurring and to take action at an early stage.
- Protection – supporting and representing those with the greatest need, particularly those with care and support needs.
- Accountability – ensuring transparency in delivering safeguarding, with clear roles and responsibilities for everyone involved.
- Partnership – working together with local communities, agencies and services to prevent and respond to abuse and neglect.
- Proportionality – taking the least intrusive response that is appropriate to the risk presented.

The Adult Safeguarding Principles within the Adult Support and Protection (Scotland) Act 2007 (Scottish Government, 2008) are as follows:

- Consider the individuals' feelings and wishes
- Consider the views of other significant individuals such as guardians, carers or attorneys
- Consider the views of any other person with an interest in the individual's property or well-being
- Provide the individual with relevant information to enable them to participate as fully as possible in the process
- Importance of treating the individual no less favourably than any other adult (in similar/comparable situation)
- Consider the adult's characteristics and background (Scottish Government, 2008).

Who is at Risk?

Anyone can be the victim of abuse, as there may be points in their life when they could be at risk of someone taking advantage of them (JRCALC and AACE, 2022). The Social Services and Well-being (Wales) Act (2014) defines an adult at risk as an individual who is experiencing or is at risk of abuse, has needs for care and support and, because of those needs, is unable to protect themselves from the abuse (or the risk of it). The Northern Ireland Adult Safeguarding: Prevention and Protection in

CHAPTER 12 Safeguarding

Partnership policy (Northern Ireland Department of Health, 2015) defines an adult at risk of harm as an individual aged 18 or over whose exposure to harm through abuse, exploitation or neglect may be increased by their personal characteristics and/or life circumstances. The Adult Support and Protection (Scotland) Act 2007 defines adults at risk as those who are unable to manage their own well-being, property, rights or other interests; are at risk of harm and because they are affected by disability, mental disorder, illness or physical or mental infirmity, are more vulnerable to being harmed than adults who are not so affected (Scottish Government, 2008).

An individual could temporarily be at risk; for example, they could have been through a traumatic experience or be recently bereaved, they could be medically unwell and once treated no longer at risk, they could be under the influence of substances and at any given time unable to make decisions for themselves.

Adults at risk were previously referred to as 'vulnerable adults' (Mandelstam, 2009; ACT, 2022). Labelling people as 'vulnerable' is no longer the preferred terminology as it is seen as disempowering and may imply the adult invited the abuse due to their vulnerability. The language has been updated to make it clear that abuse is not linked to an individual's characteristics, but their circumstances (Care Act 2014; ACT, 2022; Starns, 2019).

When needs for care and support or personal characteristics are identified, consideration should be given to an individual's mental health and cognition, for example, whether they have a condition affecting their capacity, whether they have a learning disability, whether they are on the Autistic Spectrum, whether they misuse alcohol/substances or have a physical or sensory disability.

The Mental Capacity Act

Whether an individual has capacity can be decided using the principles of the Mental Capacity Act 2005. An individual is autonomous when they have capacity and can make decisions regarding choice, freedom of will, liberty, rights and self-governance (Nixon, 2013). Healthcare professionals must consider and respect patient autonomy with every patient encounter, as it is an important aspect of every patient interaction and the basis of their decision making (Nixon, 2013).

Healthcare professionals need an awareness of best interests decisions. These are decisions taken on behalf of a person lacking capacity and must always be taken in that person's best interests. When making a best interests decision, practitioners should include the individual in the process (where possible), identify all relevant circumstances to the decision being made, ascertain a person's views and avoid discrimination. Practitioners must assess whether the individual may regain capacity and they must not make assumptions about a person's quality of life, avoid restriction of rights and should consult others if possible (Mental Capacity Act 2005). Nelson et al. (2019) suggest 'making safeguarding personal' which facilitates a person-led approach that focuses on outcomes, engages individuals and enables involvement, ultimately improving well-being and safety.

Box 12.1 Places Where Abuse and Neglect Can Happen.

Where does abuse and neglect happen?

- Residential or day care provision
- Private dwelling
- Vehicles (private or public transport)
- Hospitals
- Public buildings
- Public places such as parks, sporting/recreational facilities, clubs
- In the workplace
- In educational settings

Perpetrators

An abuser/perpetrator may be anyone from any background, religion, race, gender, profession and may be a family member, friend, colleague, stranger, professional or carer (JRCALC and AACE, 2022). All a perpetrator needs to cause harm is access to an adult at risk and the opportunity to take advantage of them (Starns, 2019). Box 12.1 highlights places where abuse and neglect can happen. Understanding that perpetrators are everywhere and can be anyone deepens our awareness of the breadth of safeguarding situations. It is also worth noting that physical contact is not necessary for all types of abuse; for example, scams which only need internet/phone contact are considered financial abuse. Everyone should be aware that research suggests that most perpetrators are someone close to the victim. Some situations will have more than one perpetrator and more than one victim; for example, a culture of emotional abuse by staff in an institution where everyone thinks it is acceptable.

Types of Abuse

There are different categories of abuse which professionals should be aware of to help identify specific concerns. Often there is more than one type of abuse occurring simultaneously and although recognition of the type of abuse is beneficial, uncertainty of the type of abuse should not prohibit reporting concerns. Safeguarding concerns can still be shared when the reporter is unsure of the type of abuse occurring. The relevant local authority will make determinations based on their further enquiries. Below is further information on some common forms of abuse.

Physical Abuse

This is when a perpetrator deliberately physically hurts an individual; this can include hitting, slapping, poisoning, punching, sedation, kicking, burning or biting. Inappropriate physical restraint, such as tying to a chair and the administration of someone else's medication, is also physical abuse.

CHAPTER 12   Safeguarding

Sexual Abuse

This is enticing or forcing an individual to take part in sexual activities. Adult sexual abuse refers to sexual assaults or sexual acts which the adult could not consent to or was pressured into consenting to. Sexual abuse can be contact (penetrative/non-penetrative acts) or non-contact (showing the victim images/videos or grooming from a distance using the internet).

Psychological Abuse

This is also known as emotional abuse. This harm can include coercive control, abandonment, threats of violence, isolation, humiliation, verbal or racial abuse. This abuse is often present with other types of abuse and is no less harmful. Survivors have described emotional abuse as leaving 'invisible wounds' which can take significant time to heal. Witnessing the abuse of others is also considered psychological abuse; this is particularly important should professionals become aware of children living in a household where domestic abuse is occurring or has occurred. These children are being subjected to emotional abuse and these concerns must be reported.

Neglect

This is an act of omission or a failure to meet needs in a way that is likely to impact on health or well-being. A failure to protect an adult at risk from danger is also considered neglect, for example, an adult at risk requiring one to one care being left alone and consequently hurting themselves. Neglect is often witnessed where there is poor personal hygiene, squalid/dangerous living conditions or a failure to seek appropriate health needs in a timely manner. Wilful neglect refers to intentional neglect by a care worker in England and Wales and is considered an offence under the Criminal Justice and Courts Act 2015. Neglect is not always intentional but can be the result of families struggling to cope with changing circumstances.

An example of this could be an older couple living independently, where one partner gradually becomes unwell. One of them has Alzheimer's disease, which impairs their ability to manage daily self-care, while the other has long-standing mobility issues that prevent them from providing adequate support with personal hygiene and meal preparation. Despite their growing difficulties, the couple continues to struggle in silence, driven by their determination to remain independent, a lack of awareness about available assistance and the fear of being separated if they acknowledge their challenges. In this scenario, both individuals are at risk due to their care and support needs, but one is unintentionally neglecting the other by not seeking additional help. This situation is common in emergency and urgent care, where a crisis often forces a request for assistance. It is crucial that practitioners recognise these situations and report them to ensure ongoing support.

Financial Abuse

This is very prevalent in adults, especially the older adult. It can present in a variety of ways, such as scamming, fraud, theft, restricting a person's access to their own funds and having undue influence on someone's financial affairs. Practitioners should be aware of a lasting power of attorney, a legal document which allows adults to appoint other(s) to help make decisions on their behalf. In England and Wales, only when a power of attorney for financial decisions is in place can someone make those decisions on behalf of someone else and there are different processes involved in Northern Ireland and Scotland.

Domestic Abuse

This can involve any or all of the four main categories of abuse. The Domestic Abuse Act 2021 defines domestic abuse as

> 'any incident or pattern of incidents of controlling, coercive, threatening behaviour, violence or abuse between those aged 16 or over who are, or have been, intimate partners or family members regardless of gender or sexuality. The abuse can encompass, but is not limited to psychological, physical, sexual, financial, emotional'.

Organisational Abuse

This is poor care or neglect which happens within a specific care setting. Most people think of it as only happening in nursing homes, care homes and hospitals, but it can also occur in private dwellings where care is provided. This type of abuse is usually not the result of one individual, but an organisational failing. One example of this is if a medication error occurs within a nursing home and an individual receives another residents' medication. Although one staff member made the error, which could have been an isolated incident, that staff member may have received poor training (causing ongoing/repeated incidents), they may be poorly supervised or unsupported by management and, when the error occurred, there may have been staffing issues placing undue pressure on that individual staff member (Davies, 2019).

Well-Being and Person-Centred Care

Spreadbury and Hubbard (2020) state it is important to consider well-being during every contact with an individual.

Some practical things to consider regarding well-being are:

- Does the individual have a system in place to raise the alarm if they fell?
- Do they have a system in place where emergency services can gain access to the property in an emergency?
- Do they have the necessary adjustments to their property to support them living independently?
- Do they require a walking stick or walking frame?
- Are they able to mobilise to the bathroom?
- Do they have access to a bathroom during the day?
- Are they able to complete personal hygiene tasks themselves?

- Do they need their chair/sofa lifted with risers to aid with standing?
- Do they need any adaptations?
- Are there any trip hazards in the property?
- Are they able to go shopping for food or prepare food themselves?

According to the Care Act 2014, 'well-being' is the term used for a wide range of things, such as:

- Personal dignity (including treating the individual with respect)
- Physical and mental health and emotional well-being
- Protection from abuse and neglect
- Control by the individual over day-to-day life (including over care and support provided to the individual and the way in which it is provided)
- Participation in work, education, training or recreation
- Social and economic well-being
- Domestic, family and personal relationships
- Suitability of living accommodation
- The individual's contribution to society.

A person-centred approach is where professionals and organisations place the person at the centre of their own decision making to maintain their well-being (Barnett, 2019). This can often be by supportive measures to ensure relocation back into family and community life by limiting risk and promoting choice, safety and well-being (Barnett, 2019). Practical considerations when attending an older person at home would include consideration of their safety, ADLs and their mobility (more detail can be found in Chapter 7: Activities of Daily Living).

Safeguarding and Legislation

Local authorities have statutory powers, alongside the police, to make enquiries into any reported safeguarding concerns. Concerns regarding the possible neglect or abuse of an adult at risk are made under section 126 of the Social Services and Well-being (Wales) Act 2014, the Adult Support and Protection (Scotland) Act 2007 and section 42 of the Care Act 2014 in England. At the time of writing Northern Ireland has the policy 'Adult Safeguarding: Prevention and Protection in Partnership' (2015) and is discussing the Adult Safeguarding Bill (2015) (Northern Ireland Department of Health, 2015).

All UK safeguarding legislation and policy defines a specific group of individuals deemed as adults that require protection, usually due to their inability to protect themselves because of disability or illness (Spreadbury and Hubbard, 2020). The specific elements and expectations of each piece of legislation are different. It is imperative that clinicians responsible for making safeguarding reports, including paramedics and other community-based teams, familiarise themselves with the relevant legal framework for their nation, profession and organisation (Spreadbury and Hubbard, 2020).

Many areas of UK legislation impact safeguarding practice. There is legislation that relates to specialist elements of safeguarding practice, such as the Female Genital Mutilation Act 2003, and there is legislation that the police utilise for criminal offences, for example, sexual abuse is convicted in accordance with the Sexual Offences Act 2003. All UK nations now have a specific act which is dedicated to domestic abuse. Wales was first with the Violence Against Women, Domestic Abuse and Sexual Violence (Wales) Act 2015; Scotland followed with the Domestic Abuse (Scotland) Act 2018; England has the Domestic Abuse Act 2021 and there is the Domestic Abuse and Civil Proceedings Act (Northern Ireland) 2021. These all make it clear that coercive and controlling behaviour is illegal across the UK.

Of note recently is the addition of a new criminal offence in England and Wales called 'non-fatal strangulation or suffocation'. This offence has been created due to the introduction of the Domestic Abuse Act 2021 which amends the Serious Crime Act 2015, adding sections 75A and 75B (Home Office, 2022). This is relevant for safeguarding practitioners who attend instances of domestic abuse during an emergency care episode. An abuser affecting an individual's ability to breathe could be evidence of escalating behaviours. Strangulation is one method that a perpetrator will use to inflict a terrifying ordeal upon their victim, instilling fear by using power and control. Strangulation-causing asphyxiation is the second most common technique in domestic homicides with female victims (England and Wales only) (Home Office, 2022).

All professionals involved in health and social care must consider human rights as they are found within national standards and codes/guides of conduct. Advocating an individual's human rights promotes professional accountability within the service in which you work and ensures service users are protected. Professionals must report any witnessed human rights violations as it is a professional obligation (Health Information and Quality Authority, 2019). Rights which an older person may need help with are:

- The right to be safe
- The right to privacy
- The right to be treated with dignity and respect
- The right to be involved in decisions about their own life
- The right to live free from abuse and exploitation
- The right to an adequate standard of living
- The right to the highest possible standard of physical and mental health
- The right to social security
- The right to participate in cultural life and to enjoy the benefits of scientific progress.

CHAPTER 12 Safeguarding

Safeguarding in Emergency and Urgent Care

Safeguarding is part of mandatory training for most workers within NHS trusts and the wider health and social care settings. It is a key part of all patient interactions and has a legislative basis in England, Scotland, Wales and policy in Northern Ireland. This places a duty upon all healthcare professionals and all staff providing care and support to service users to consider their patient's well-being. The level of training will vary depending on position and organisation, it may be an online learning package or a half or full-day face-to-face session.

Professional registration ensures that different professionals within healthcare settings are accountable to a professional governing body, which ensure all individuals within these professions are fit to practice and can effectively safeguard patients (Nixon, 2013). The Health and Care Professions Council standards of conduct, performance and ethics include information particularly related to safeguarding (2018). There are many non-registrants within the health and social care setting who still have safeguarding responsibilities even though they have no regulatory professional body. There are also a range of organisations across the UK who monitor and inspect care services to ensure the quality and safety of services which includes safeguarding adults at risk. There are often specific parts of policies that refer to carers as they have a range of safeguarding roles. Their position may leave them vulnerable to harm themselves, they may raise concerns or be the abusers (Somerset Adults Safeguarding Board, 2019).

A key element of safeguarding is also education and increasing public awareness of the signs, symptoms, indicators and dangers of abuse and neglect. Effective training is essential to ensure safeguarding practice is current and of good quality (Dawson, 2021). For many years it has been known that prehospital and community professionals are in a unique position to safeguard as they have access to information others do not; they are welcomed into homes at unexpected times. This means they have a view of the natural home environment meaning they may witness things that may have changed by the time others visit (for example, social workers) (Greaves et al., 1997). Professionals working prehospitally are also privy to the 'initial story'. This initial story is critical as an inconsistent history is a key indicator of physical abuse (Greaves et al., 1997). Further to this, it is crucial that healthcare professionals do not underestimate the value of the knowledge they have, as no one else has witnessed, heard, smelt or been told what they have in that patient interaction. Healthcare professionals should consider safeguarding as a jigsaw puzzle and that their information is one jigsaw piece; that piece could be the crucial final piece that the local authority may require to see the overall picture and could make all the difference to ensure the safety of an adult at risk.

Professional Curiosity

It is often very difficult to identify abuse and neglect as individuals experiencing it may not disclose their abuse and may only provide insight through their behaviour or body language (Leeds Local Authority, 2022). Being professionally curious when talking to service users, practising 'respectful uncertainty' and being inquisitive to explore a situation further, rather than accepting everything at face value, can reveal safeguarding concerns (Leeds Local Authority, 2022). There is no expectation to investigate concerns, but to ask appropriate questions. Professional curiosity can also reveal disguised compliance. A multitude of published adult case reviews evidence instances where a lack of professional curiosity and disguised compliance delayed safeguarding actions being taken and the individuals came to further harm as a result (Lancashire Safeguarding, 2022). Respectful uncertainty is critically evaluating the information provided to ensure the safety of our patients (Lord Laming, 2003).

Conclusion

Some healthcare professionals state that they have worked within the healthcare service for years and never come across safeguarding concerns. Based upon the prevalence of abuse and neglect it is far more likely that those healthcare professionals have not recognised the safeguarding concerns when they came across them. It is important to remember that everyone has the right to live free from abuse and neglect. Some adults at risk, including older adults, are unable to protect themselves from harm and require support. Anyone can be an adult at risk during their lifetime and harm could happen anywhere at any time. Safeguarding adults is an essential consideration of every patient interaction (they could be an adult at risk). National legislation and local/organisational reporting procedures and policies must be followed. All an abuser/perpetrator needs to continue causing harm is for nothing to change – reporting a concern is taking decisive action to prevent or stop harm and most importantly, reporting safeguarding concerns is everyone's responsibility – do not assume it has been done by someone else.

Questions

1. Are you aware of your local safeguarding procedures?
2. Think of a recent incident in which you considered a safeguarding report. How would the knowledge in this chapter change your safeguarding report approach if you encountered the same situation again?
3. How do safeguarding presentations differ for older people? What types of abuse would you need to explore in further detail?

Further Resources

- Safeguarding Board for Northern Ireland.: https://www.safeguardingni.org
- Scottish Government, Policy: Social Care, Adult support and protection: https://www.gov.scot/policies/social-care/adult-support-and-protection/#:~:text=All%20adults%20at%20risk%20of,mental%20disorder
- The Care Act 2014: https://www.legislation.gov.uk/ukpga/2014/23/contents
- Wales Safeguarding Procedure. Social Care Wales: https://www.google.com/url?sa=t&source=web&rct=j&opi=89978449&url=https://socialcare.wales/cms-assets/documents/2020-All-Wales-Basic-Safeguarding-Awareness-Wales-Safeguarding-Pack.pptx&ved=2ahUKEwinvvyT9t6HAxVdVkEAHZTUL2EQFnoECBUQAQ&usg=AOvVaw2loEf30EqY96vw9sy3oOF6

CHAPTER 12 Safeguarding

References

Ann Craft Trust (ACT) (2022). Safeguarding Adults Definitions. Available at: https://www.anncrafttrust.org/resources/safeguarding-adults-at-risk-definitions/#:~:text=%E2%80%9CAdult%20safeguarding%E2%80%9D%20is%20working%20with,of%20all%20adults%20is%20ensured [accessed 4th September 2022].

Barnett D (2019). *The Straightforward Guide to Safeguarding Adults: From getting the basics right to applying the care act and criminal investigations*. London: Jessica Kingsley Publishers.

Care Act 2014. UK Public General Acts, c. 23. Available at: https://www.legislation.gov.uk/ukpga/2014/23/contents/enacted [accessed 1st June 2024].

Criminal Justice and Courts Act 2015, 20–21. Available at: https://www.legislation.gov.uk/ukpga/2015/2/contents [accessed 12th April 2024].

Davies E (2019). What is institutional abuse? Definitions, signs and symptoms. Ann Craft Trust. Available at: https://www.anncrafttrust.org/institutional-abuse-definitions-signs-symptoms/ [accessed 27th September 2023].

Dawson B (2021). *Adult Safeguarding: Could we do better? A trainer's perspective* (1st edition). Gloucester: The Choir Press.

Domestic Abuse (Scotland) Act 2018, asp. 5. Available at: https://www.legislation.gov.uk/asp/2018/5/contents/enacted [accessed 1st June 2024].

Domestic Abuse Act 2021, c. 17. Available at: https://www.legislation.gov.uk/ukpga/2021/17/contents/enacted [accessed 12th April 2024].

Domestic Abuse and Civil Proceedings Act (Northern Ireland) 2021, c. 2. Available at: https://www.legislation.gov.uk/nia/2021/2/contents [accessed 1st June 2024].

Female Genital Mutilation Act 2003, c. 31. Available at: https://www.legislation.gov.uk/ukpga/2003/31/contents [accessed 1st June 2024].

Greaves I, Hodgetts T, Porter K (1997). *Emergency Care*. London: W.B. Saunders.

Health and Care Professions Council (2018). *Standards of Conduct, Performance and Ethics*. Available at: https://www.hcpc-uk.org/standards/standards-of-conduct-performance-and-ethics/ [accessed 4th September 2024].

Health Information and Quality Authority (2019). Guidance on a human rights-based approach in health and social care services. HIQA and Safeguarding Ireland. Available at: https://www.hiqa.ie/sites/default/files/2019-11/Human-Rights-Based-Approach-Guide.PDF [accessed 4th September 2024].

Home Office (2022). Strangulation and suffocation policy paper. Available at: https://www.gov.uk/government/publications/domestic-abuse-bill-2020-factsheets/strangulation-and-suffocation#will-this-new-offence-apply-across-the-uk:%20Home%20Office [accessed 1st June 2024].

Joint Royal Colleges Ambulance Liaison Committee (JRCALC) and Association of Ambulance Chief Executives (AACE) (2022). *JRCALC Clinical Guidelines 2022*. Bridgwater: Class Professional Publishing.

Lancashire Safeguarding (2022). 7-minute briefing: COVID-19 professional curiosity. Blackburn with Darwen, Blackpool and Lancashire Children's Safeguarding Assurance Partnership and Adult Safeguarding Boards. Available at: https://www.lancashiresafeguarding.org.uk/media/19220/CV-19-7mb-Professional-Curiosty.pdf [accessed 25th September 2023].

Leeds Local Authority (2022). One Minute Guide: Professional curiosity. Available at: https://www.leeds.gov.uk/one-minute-guides/professional-curiosity [accessed 1st October 2024].

Lord Laming (2003). *The Victoria Climbié Enquiry*. Norwich: TSO.

Mandelstam M (2009). *Safeguarding Vulnerable Adults and the Law*. London: Jessica Kingsley Publishers.

References

Mental Capacity Act 2005, c. 9. Available at: https://www.legislation.gov.uk/ukpga/2005/9/contents [accessed 1st June 2024].

Nelson P, et al. (2019). Making safeguarding personal temperature check – Doncaster MBC. Available at: from https://shura.shu.ac.uk/24671/3/Nelson-MakingSafeguardingPersonal%28AM%29.pdf [accessed 1st June 2024].

Nixon V (2013). *Professional Practice in Paramedic, Emergency and Urgent Care*. Chichester: Wiley Blackwell.

Northern Ireland Department of Health (2015). Adult safeguarding: Prevention and protection in partnership. Available at: https://www.health-ni.gov.uk/publications/adult-safeguarding-prevention-and-protection-partnership-key-documents

Scottish Government (2008). Adult Support and Protection (Scotland) Act 2007. Available at: https://www.gov.scot/publications/adult-support-protection-scotland-act-2007-short-introduction-part-1-act/ [accessed 1st June 2024].

Serious Crime Act 2015, c. 9. Available at: https://www.legislation.gov.uk/ukpga/2015/9/contents/enacted [accessed 1st June 2024].

Sexual Offences Act 2003, c. 42. Available at: https://www.legislation.gov.uk/ukpga/2003/42/contents [accessed 1st June 2024].

Social Services and Well-being (Wales) Act 2014, anaw 4. Available at: https://www.legislation.gov.uk/anaw/2014/4/contents [accessed 1st June 2024].

Somerset Safeguarding Adults Board (2019). Safeguarding adults multi-agency policy. Available at: https://nhssomerset.nhs.uk/wp-content/uploads/sites/2/20190625-FINAL-Joint-Safeguarding-Adults-Policy-Somerset.pdf [accessed 1st June 2024].

Spreadbury K, Hubbard R (2020). *The Adult Safeguarding Practice Handbook*. Bristol: Policy Press.

Starns B (2019). *Safeguarding Adults Together Under the Care Act 2014*. St Albans: Critical Publishing Ltd.

Violence against Women, Domestic Abuse and Sexual Violence (Wales) Act 2015, anaw 3. Available at: https://www.legislation.gov.uk/anaw/2015/3/contents/enacted [accessed 1st June 2024].

Welsh Government (2019). Wales safeguarding procedures. Available at: https://safeguarding.wales/en/ [accessed 8th June 2024].

Index

Page numbers followed by *f* denote figures; those followed by *t* denote tables and those followed by *b* denote boxes

4 'A's Test (4AT), 36, 40

A

Abuse,
    domestic, 193
    financial, 192–193
    legislation, 194–195
    neglect, 192
    organisational, 193
    overview and definition, 188
    perpetrators of, 191
    physical, 191
    psychological, 192
    sexual, 192
    'who is at risk', 189–190
ACP. *See* Advanced clinical practitioner
Activities of daily living, 7, 103–115
    causes and symptoms, 106–107
    environment, 113–114
    functional assessment, 107–112
    motivation, 114
    risk assessment, 114–115
    sudden onset immobility, 106
    walking aids, 112–113
Acute illness, 127
Acute interstitial nephritis, 60, 60*t*
Acute tubular injury, 60*t*
Adaptive homeostasis theory, 8
ADLs. *See* Activities of daily living
ADRs. *See* Adverse Drug Reactions
Advance care planning, 44, 160
Advanced clinical practitioners, 23

Advanced Trauma Life Support, 143, 146
Adverse Drug Reactions, 87–89, 87*t*–88*t*
AFib. *See* Atrial fibrillation
Ageing
    biological theories of, 7–9
    physiology of, 11–14
    psychological theories of, 10–11
    sociological theories of, 9–10
Ageism, 21–22
Agitation, 166–167
    non-pharmacological management, 167
    pharmacological management, 167
Airway and cervical spine, trauma, 147–148
Alcohol and non-prescription medications, 129
Alzheimer's disease, 68
Anticholinergic burden (ACB) calculator, 95*t*
Anxiety, 71–74, 166–167
    assessing, 72
    key considerations, 72–73
    legal/ethical considerations, 73
    management, 73–74
    non-pharmacological management, 167
    pharmacological management, 167
Aortic stenosis, 54–55
Asthma, 51–53
    action plan, 51*t*
    primary care management of, 51
    risk factors for, 51
ATLS. *See* Advanced Trauma Life Support
Atrial fibrillation, 55–57
    causes of, 56*b*
    referral for patients with, 56*t*

Index

B

BADLs. *See* Basic ADLs
Balance, 124
Basic ADLs, 106
Behavioural theory, 11
Biological theories of ageing, 7–9
    adaptive homeostasis theory, 8
    epigenetic clock theory, 8–9
    free radical theory, 7–8
    genetic theory, 8
Breathing, 148–149
Breathlessness, 165–166
    non-pharmacological management, 166
    pharmacological management, 166
Burns, 150–151

C

Capacity, 69
Cardiac events, 124
Cardiovascular system, changes in, 12
Care Act 2014, 176–180, 176b, 177b
Care home, 181
Carers, 176–177
    Case studies
    falls, 119–121
    frailty, 31–33, 38t
    long-term conditions, 49–50
    major trauma, 141–143
    mental health and cognition, 65–67
    palliative and end-of-life care, 155–157
    person-centred communication, 19
    polypharmacy, 81–82
    safeguarding, 185–188
    social care, 173–175
Catastrophic haemorrhage, 147
CFS. *See* Clinical Frailty Scale
CGA. *See* Comprehensive Geriatric Assessment
Chronic obstructive pulmonary disease, 51–53, 52f, 51t
Chronic pain, 62
Clinical Frailty Scale, 35, 35t, 37f
Cognition, 124–125
Cognitive theories, 10
Communication. *See* Person-centred communication
    breakdowns, 20–21
    with other healthcare providers, 27–28
    skills, 26t–27t
    underdeveloped skills, 24
Comprehensive Geriatric Assessment, 42–44, 43f
CAM. *See* Confusion Assessment Method
Confusion Assessment Method, 40
COPD. *See* Chronic obstructive pulmonary disease
Corticosteroid treatment, side effects of, 53b
Crystalline nephropathies, 60t
Culture, 24–25

D

Dehydration, 125
Deliberate self-harm
    assessment, 74
    legal/ethical considerations, 74–75
    management, 75
Delirium, 39–41, 71
    assessment and diagnosis, 40
    management of, 41
Dementia, 68–71
    acute medical illness in patients diagnosed with, 71
    assessment, 68–69
    key considerations, 69
    legal/ethical considerations, 69–70
    management, 70–71
Depression, 71–74
    assessing, 72
    key considerations, 72–73
    legal/ethical considerations, 73
    management, 73, 74b
Dermatological changes, physiology of ageing, 13
Determinants of well-being and health theory, 9–10
Diabetes, management of, 57
Diagnostic and Statistical Manual of Mental Disorders (DSM-5), 40
Dizziness, 126
Domestic abuse, 193
Dynamic balance, 109, 124

E

ECG. *See* Electrocardiogram
eFI. *See* Electronic Frailty Index

Index

Page numbers followed by *f* denote figures; those followed by *t* denote tables and those followed by *b* denote boxes

4 'A's Test (4AT), 36, 40

A

Abuse,
    domestic, 193
    financial, 192–193
    legislation, 194–195
    neglect, 192
    organisational, 193
    overview and definition, 188
    perpetrators of, 191
    physical, 191
    psychological, 192
    sexual, 192
    'who is at risk', 189–190
ACP. *See* Advanced clinical practitioner
Activities of daily living, 7, 103–115
    causes and symptoms, 106–107
    environment, 113–114
    functional assessment, 107–112
    motivation, 114
    risk assessment, 114–115
    sudden onset immobility, 106
    walking aids, 112–113
Acute illness, 127
Acute interstitial nephritis, 60, 60*t*
Acute tubular injury, 60*t*
Adaptive homeostasis theory, 8
ADLs. *See* Activities of daily living
ADRs. *See* Adverse Drug Reactions
Advance care planning, 44, 160
Advanced clinical practitioners, 23
Advanced Trauma Life Support, 143, 146
Adverse Drug Reactions, 87–89, 87*t*–88*t*
AFib. *See* Atrial fibrillation
Ageing
    biological theories of, 7–9
    physiology of, 11–14
    psychological theories of, 10–11
    sociological theories of, 9–10
Ageism, 21–22
Agitation, 166–167
    non-pharmacological management, 167
    pharmacological management, 167
Airway and cervical spine, trauma, 147–148
Alcohol and non-prescription medications, 129
Alzheimer's disease, 68
Anticholinergic burden (ACB) calculator, 95*t*
Anxiety, 71–74, 166–167
    assessing, 72
    key considerations, 72–73
    legal/ethical considerations, 73
    management, 73–74
    non-pharmacological management, 167
    pharmacological management, 167
Aortic stenosis, 54–55
Asthma, 51–53
    action plan, 51*t*
    primary care management of, 51
    risk factors for, 51
ATLS. *See* Advanced Trauma Life Support
Atrial fibrillation, 55–57
    causes of, 56*b*
    referral for patients with, 56*t*

Index

B

BADLs. *See* Basic ADLs
Balance, 124
Basic ADLs, 106
Behavioural theory, 11
Biological theories of ageing, 7–9
    adaptive homeostasis theory, 8
    epigenetic clock theory, 8–9
    free radical theory, 7–8
    genetic theory, 8
Breathing, 148–149
Breathlessness, 165–166
    non-pharmacological management, 166
    pharmacological management, 166
Burns, 150–151

C

Capacity, 69
Cardiac events, 124
Cardiovascular system, changes in, 12
Care Act 2014, 176–180, 176b, 177b
Care home, 181
Carers, 176–177
    Case studies
    falls, 119–121
    frailty, 31–33, 38t
    long-term conditions, 49–50
    major trauma, 141–143
    mental health and cognition, 65–67
    palliative and end-of-life care, 155–157
    person-centred communication, 19
    polypharmacy, 81–82
    safeguarding, 185–188
    social care, 173–175
Catastrophic haemorrhage, 147
CFS. *See* Clinical Frailty Scale
CGA. *See* Comprehensive Geriatric Assessment
Chronic obstructive pulmonary disease, 51–53, 52f, 51t
Chronic pain, 62
Clinical Frailty Scale, 35, 35t, 37f
Cognition, 124–125
Cognitive theories, 10
Communication. *See* Person-centred communication
    breakdowns, 20–21
    with other healthcare providers, 27–28
    skills, 26t–27t
    underdeveloped skills, 24
Comprehensive Geriatric Assessment, 42–44, 43f
CAM. *See* Confusion Assessment Method
Confusion Assessment Method, 40
COPD. *See* Chronic obstructive pulmonary disease
Corticosteroid treatment, side effects of, 53b
Crystalline nephropathies, 60t
Culture, 24–25

D

Dehydration, 125
Deliberate self-harm
    assessment, 74
    legal/ethical considerations, 74–75
    management, 75
Delirium, 39–41, 71
    assessment and diagnosis, 40
    management of, 41
Dementia, 68–71
    acute medical illness in patients diagnosed with, 71
    assessment, 68–69
    key considerations, 69
    legal/ethical considerations, 69–70
    management, 70–71
Depression, 71–74
    assessing, 72
    key considerations, 72–73
    legal/ethical considerations, 73
    management, 73, 74b
Dermatological changes, physiology of ageing, 13
Determinants of well-being and health theory, 9–10
Diabetes, management of, 57
Diagnostic and Statistical Manual of Mental Disorders (DSM-5), 40
Dizziness, 126
Domestic abuse, 193
Dynamic balance, 109, 124

E

ECG. *See* Electrocardiogram
eFI. *See* Electronic Frailty Index

Index

Electrocardiogram, 55
Electronic Frailty Index, 36
Emotional abuse, 192
Emotional theory, 10
Environment, 113–114, 130
Epigenetic clock theory, 8–9
Ethical considerations
    of anxiety, 73
    dementia, 69–70
    deliberate self-harm, 74–75
    depression, 73
    falls, 134–135
Executive functioning, 106
Extrinsic factors, falls, 129–130

F

Falls
    case study, 119–121
    clinical investigations, 132–133
    complications, 130–132
    defined, 121
    ethical considerations, 134–135
    extrinsic factors, 129–130
    frailty syndrome, 121
    functional assessments, 133
    intrinsic factors, 124–129
    older person who has fallen, 122–124
Fear of falling, 125
Feet, falls, 125
Financial abuse, 192–193
FiND Questionnaire, 36
FIST. *See* Function in sitting test
Footwear, falls, 129
Fragility fractures, 131
Frailty, 31–46, 125
    applying tool, 36–39
    case study, 31–33, 38*t*
    defining, 34
    introduction, 33–34
    measurement and screening tools, 35–36
    socioeconomic factors, 34
    syndromes, 34, 39–42
Frames, 112
Free radical theory, 7–8
FRESH-Screening tool, 36
Function in sitting test, 107

G

Gait cycle, 109, 109*f*, 110*t*, 129
Gait speed test, 111
Gastrointestinal system, physiology of ageing, 12–13
General practitioner assessment of cognition, 69
Genetic theory, 8
Genitourinary system, physiology of ageing, 13
Gold Standards Framework, 161
GPCOG. *See* General practitioner assessment of cognition
GSF. *See* Gold Standards Framework

H

Haematological system, physiology of ageing, 11–12
Handrails, 113
Head cancer, 62*b*
Head injuries, in older people, 130–131, 130*t*
Health, social determinants of, 9*f*
Heart failure, 53, 54*t*
Heartlands Elderly Care Trauma & Ongoing Recovery Programme (HECTOR), 143, 147
HECTOR. *See* Heartlands Elderly Care Trauma & Ongoing Recovery Programme
Homeostasis changes, physiology of ageing, 11
Homeostenosis, 11
Human development, stage theories of, 10–11
Hyperactive delirium, 40
Hypotension, 125
Hypothermia, 132
Hypothyroidism, 58

I

IADLs. *See* Instrumental ADLs
Iatrogenic acute kidney injury, 60, 60*t*
Immobility, frailty syndrome, 41
Immunosenescence, 11
Incontinence, 127
    frailty syndrome, 41–42
Instrumental ADLs, 106
Intrinsic factors, falls, 124–129

Index

J

Jargon, person-centred communication, 23–24

L

Lighting, falls, 129
Loneliness, 34, 74b
Long lie, 131
Long-term conditions
    aortic stenosis, 54–55
    asthma and, 51–53
    atrial fibrillation, 55–57, 56b, 56t
    case study, 49–50
    chronic obstructive pulmonary disease, 51–53
    chronic pain, 62
    diabetes, 55
    heart failure, 53, 54t
    iatrogenic acute kidney injury, 60
    introduction, 50
    malignancy, 61, 62b
    osteoarthritis, 60–61
    Parkinson's disease, 59–60
    stroke/transient ischaemic attack, 58–59
    thyroid, 58
Low body mass index, 127
LTCs. See Long term conditions

M

Major trauma
    abdominal injuries, 151–152
    age differences, 144–145
    approaches, 147–150
    burns, 150–151
    case study, 141–143
    circulation, 149
    data patterns in, 145–146
    defined, 144
    disability, 149–150
    exposure, 150
    nature of, 143
    pain management, 152
    pelvis and hip injuries, 151
Malignancy, 61, 62b
Medicine, adverse drug reactions, 87–89, 87t–88t
Medicine reviews
    medicines reconciliation and history, 91–92
    need, 92
    principles of, 92–97
    tools, 93t
Medicines reconciliation, 91–92
Mental Capacity Act 2005, 69, 70b, 190
Mental health and cognition
    anxiety, 71–74
    case study, 65–67
    deliberate self-harm, 74–75
    delirium, 71
    dementia, 68–71
    depression, 71–74
    introduction, 68
    schizophrenia, 75–76
Microaggressions, 23
Motivation, activities of daily living, 114
Motor symptoms, Parkinson's disease, 59–60
Muscle weakness, 127–128
Musculoskeletal system, 13

N

National Early Warning Score 2, 36
Nausea and vomiting
    non-pharmacological management, 168
    pharmacological management, 168
Near-syncope, 122
Neck cancer, 62b
Neck of femur (NOF), 151
Neglect, 192
Neurogenic OH, 126
Neurological conditions, falls, 128
Neurological system, physiology of ageing, 12
NEWS2. See National Early Warning Score 2
Non-motor symptoms, Parkinson's disease, 59–60
Non-neurogenic OH, 126

O

OA. See Osteoarthritis
Organisational abuse, 193
Osteoarthritis, 60–61

Index

feature of, 60
multidisciplinary approach, 61f

P

Pain, 128, 164
  non-pharmacological management, 165
  pharmacological management, 165
Palliative and end-of-life care
  assessment, 163
  case study, 155–157
  difficult conversations, 163–164
  illness trajectories and, 162f
  introduction, 158
  shared decision making, 163–164
  symptoms in, 164–169
Parkinson's disease, 59–60
Patient, recognising dying, 161–163
Perpetrators, 191
Person-centred approach, 194
Person-centred communication
  ageism, 21–22
  age-related changes, 24–25
  breakdowns in, 20–21
  case study, 19
  components of, 26, 26t–27t
  cultural differences, 24–25
  introduction, 20
  jargon, 23–24
  lack of provider commitment, 22–23
  with other healthcare providers, 27–28
  strategy, 26t–27t
  underdeveloped skills, 24
Pharmacokinetics principles, 84f
Physical abuse, 191
Physiology of ageing, 11–13
  cardiovascular changes, 12
  dermatological changes, 13
  gastrointestinal changes, 12–13
  genitourinary system, 13
  haematological changes, 11–12
  homeostasis changes, 11
  musculoskeletal system, 13
  neurological changes, 12
  renal changes, 13
  respiratory changes, 12
  vision, hearing, taste and smell changes, 13–14

Polypharmacy
  defined, 83
  disease, 90
  introduction, 83
  medicine, 87–90, 87t–88t
  patient, 84–87
  steps, 92–97
Postural orthostatic tachycardia syndrome, 126
POTS. *See* Postural orthostatic tachycardia syndrome
Prescribing cascade, 88–89, 89f
Pressure wounds, 131
Pre-syncope, 126
Professional curiosity, 196–197
Psychological abuse, 192
Psychological theories of ageing
  behavioural theory, 11
  cognitive theories, 10
  emotional theory, 10
  human development, stage theories of, 10–11

R

Renal system, physiology of ageing, 13
Respiratory secretions
  non-pharmacological management, 169
  pharmacological management, 169
Respiratory system, physiology of ageing, 12
Rhabdomyolysis, 132
Risk, 189–190

S

Safeguarding
  in emergency and urgent care, 196
  introduction, 188
  and legislation, 194–195
  principles, 188–189
Schizophrenia
  assessment, 75–76
  legal/ethical concerns, 76
  management, 76
  risks to patient safety, 76
  signs and symptoms, 75–76
Scottish Patients at Risk of Readmission and Admission (SPARRA), 36
Sexual abuse, 192
Sit-to-stand (STS) assessment, 108

Index

Social care
    assessment of needs, 177–179
    care home placements, 181
    carers and caring role, 176–177
    case study, 173–175
    choice and control, 180–181
    financial assessment, 179–180
    introduction, 175–176
Social determinants of health, 9f
Social identity theory, 21
Social isolation, 74b
Sociological theories of ageing
    determinants of well-being and health theory, 9–10
    successful ageing theory, 9
Stability, 124
Stage theories of human development, 10–11
Stairs, 112–113
Stand-to-sit (SIT) assessment, 108
Static balance, 124
Stroke, 58–59, 128
Successful ageing theory, 9
Susceptibility to side effects of medications, 41
Syncope, 122

T

Thyroid, 58
Thyroid stimulating hormone, 58
TIA. *See* Transient ischaemic attack
Timed Up and Go Test, 36
Toileting, ADLs, 108–109
Transient ischaemic attack, 58–59
TSH. *See* Thyroid stimulating hormone
TUGT. *See* Timed Up and Go Test

U

Upper limb function, 111–112

V

Vascular dementia, 68
Virchow's Triad, 55f
Vision, 13–14, 128
Vitamin D deficiencies, 128–129
Vomiting
    non-pharmacological management, 168
    pharmacological management, 168

W

Walking stick, 112
Well-being and person-centred care, 193–194